SUCCESSFUL GROWTH
AND DEVELOPMENT
IN THE DENTAL PRACTICE

SUCCESSFUL GROWTH AND DEVELOPMENT IN THE DENTAL PRACTICE

Anita Jupp

Dental Consultant and Professional Lecturer
Burlington, Ontario, Canada

1996 Silent Partners Publishing Inc.

Front cover photograph Imtek Imagineering/Masterfile.

NOTICE

The author and publishers have done all they can to ensure that the information provided in this book is in compliance with current practices and standards. As regulations and clinical practices are constantly changing, you are encouraged to check with your local governing body for advice on proper guidelines.

Printed in Canada

ISBN 1-896810-01-2

TABLE OF CONTENTS

ACKNOWLEDGEMENTS

As my career developed, I remember special people in the dental community who were supportive and who encouraged me – especially those individuals who attend my lectures. I must thank you whole heartedly.

My publisher Isabel encouraged me to write two books, one on administration and one on practice management techniques. It seemed like an impossible project but one of my team members, Sally Colosimo said *"we can do it"*. Lisa Simmons and Joan Uddenberg looked after the office while Sally and I combined our efforts – I wrote and she edited and organized.

A special thank you to those friends and colleagues who encouraged me to continue to write when I thought I couldn't.

My dream is that from my books I can give to dentists and their teams the same support and encouragement I received from others.

INTRODUCTION

*"The rung of a ladder was never meant to rest upon, but only to hold
a man's foot long enough to enable him to put the other somewhat higher."*

So wrote Thomas Henry Huxley. A statement which rings true to all those who dream of success. Becoming successful is not easy; it is a long and hard road on a path filled with obstacles, peaks and valleys. Hard work, dedication, commitment and an open mind for learning will be the keys to your success.

Welcome to my second book, which will take you to the next stage of development in dental practice management. My first book, *Dental Administration Made Easy*, was designed to introduce the basic business systems required to operate a successful dental practice: scheduling, collecting, insurance, predeterminations and communication.

Sadly, management skills are not taught at most dental schools and universities. These are learned skills, developed over a period of time. Being a leader does not come easily to most people. Leadership develops with experience and education.

The leader sets the pace and the example for the practice. Therefore, strong business skills and a positive attitude are the qualities you want to develop and pass on to your dental team. You must identify what you, the business owner and leader, want, need and expect for the business. Identification of areas you need to improve upon will also factor into your success.

As a business grows, many dentists spread themselves too thin by trying to do everything themselves or by being completely involved in all aspects of the business. It is important to retain control but it's also important to allow your team the flexibility and encouragement to assume more responsibility.

Analyze your business and yourself to allow yourself to move ahead to a more productive and harmonious level. I believe that we do not need to make big changes to make a big difference – grow gradually toward your vision of success. **Take a Chance!** As the Nike ad says, *"Just Do It"*.

Anita Jupp
March, 1996

"Achievement comes after hard work, not before."
Michaelangelo

1.

SUCCESSFUL
STAFFING

INTRODUCTION

In any type of business, your staff is a reflection of your services. If you expect to have a successful business, it is important that you have the right staff.

- Motivated with a positive attitude
- Enthusiastic
- Organized
- Competent and intelligent

Happy people work harder and as a consumer or patient, we all want to go to the type of business where we will be treated well.

Dentists tend to focus on their dentistry but they must also realize that having the right staff is just as important to the success of their business. Many dentists complain about staff and often ignore frustrations or problems, hoping they will go away. Most often, these frustrations and problems do not go away. Dealing with staffing problems is a priority.

Being happy in our personal and business lives should be a priority. Why pay someone who makes you, your patients and other team members miserable? Find staff who complement your practice philosophy, who are focused on patients and who are personable, committed employees.

In dentistry, you must ensure that you are well staffed. If not, some areas of the practice will lack follow-up and attention. If the following responsibilities are not being met, you are possibly understaffed.

- Answering the telephone efficiently (within 3 rings).
- Greeting each patient as they come through the door.
- Controlling and appointing an effective production schedule.
- Follow-up with treatment to be completed.
- Follow-up with predeterminations and collection calls.

- Discussing fees with patients.
- Issuing a receipt to each and every patient.
- Preparing written financial arrangements.
- Preparing and making bank deposits.
- Preparing outgoing mail.
- Confirming appointments.
- Sorting incoming mail.
- Answering any and all patient inquiries related to treatment, fees, etc.
- Maintaining organized and effective business systems.
- Sterilization of instruments and following up on lab work.

If these or any other areas are neglected, your practice will suffer. It is extremely important to have the correct number of staff members to handle all of the daily responsibilities.

NETWORKING

Before resorting to a newspaper advertisement or other forms of advertising, you may wish to ask your dental team and/or friends in the dental community, if they know of anyone qualified for the position you wish to fill. Suggested candidates should be interviewed and their references checked.

DENTAL PLACEMENT AGENCIES

There are reputable agencies throughout North America who specialize in placing qualified dental professionals into suitable positions for a fee. However, by using an agency you eliminate the need to advertise and screen phone calls and resumes. Make sure that the agency you select personally interviews and checks the references of each individual they refer to you. This helps eliminate inappropriate candidates who could take up valuable time.

NEWSPAPER/JOURNAL ADVERTISEMENTS THAT WORK

When hiring a new employee, careful planning is required. As you know, high staff turnover is detrimental to your practice. Patients want to see the same friendly faces every time they visit your practice – it creates a high-trust atmosphere. For this reason, an ad that attracts applicants who fit your practice is the starting point. For example:

1. *Progressive dental practice is seeking an experienced, friendly, team-spirited dental assistant to work a five-day week in our general practice. Please forward your professional resume with cover letter c/o this newspaper, Box 1234.*

2. *Patient-centered, team-oriented dental hygienist. Is this you? If so, our large, progressive general dental practice would like to meet you to discuss our part-time position. Please send your resume with a covering letter c/o this newspaper, Box 124.*

3. *Full-time experienced business assistant required for busy, patient-centered dental office. Knowledge of computers, finances and payroll an asset. Excellent communication and friendly people skills are our top priority. Please send resume with cover letter c/o this newspaper, Box 37546.*

4. *Friendly, caring, experienced part-time dental assistant needed for our small, community-based general practice. People skills and initiative are our top priorities. We look forward to receiving your resume and cover letter c/o this newspaper, Box 865.*

5. *Full time, professional, knowledgeable, experienced dental receptionist wanted for our patient-centered, team-oriented general practice. Experience with computers, bookkeeping and business systems is necessary. Friendly and firm communication skills are a must. Some evening hours and weekends are included. We look forward to receiving your cover letter and resume. Box 3456.*

We ask for a resume with cover letter for two reasons. First, the resume will give an impression of the organizational and preparation skills of the applicant. Typed, well-spaced, neat and easy-to-read resumes will help to make your decision easier. A five-page resume is not necessary, but one filled with appropriate and applicable information is.

Second, the cover letter gives you an indication of the applicant's command of grammar, writing style and fluency. These characteristics are especially important for reception positions. The resume and cover letter are a reflection of the applicant, their motivation and their organizational abilities. As you review the resumes, set aside those with the qualifications you require for the position available. When you call to set up an interview, you will have a chance to assess the applicant's communication skills over the phone.

If your receptionist has time to screen calls from applicants, you could also place your office phone number in the ad. Keep in mind that you will receive many calls from prospective employees, which will tie up your telephone lines while your receptionist answers questions about the position. It is usually best to request a resume in order to narrow your search. Communication skills will be assessed over the telephone and at the personal interview.

THE JOB DESCRIPTION

A job description makes your interviewing process easier. Most applicants will ask what the position entails and most interviewers give only a basic description of the position. What you need to consider is not only the daily responsibilities, but also the weekly, monthly, and yearly duties of the position. A sample job description will help you to determine if the applicant is suitable for the position. It is important to also involve your team when setting the duty requirements of a new employee.

SAMPLE JOB DESCRIPTION – FULL-TIME DENTAL RECEPTIONIST

Daily Responsibilities
1. Join the team 15 minutes early for our brief morning meeting.
2. Greet incoming patients with a warm, friendly smile.
3. Productively schedule one dentist, one assistant and one hygienist.
4. Answer all incoming lines.
5. Take care of patient payments, insurance and predeterminations as required.
6. Make all computer entries (or day sheet entries) promptly.
7. Pull all patient charts for the next day for confirmation, and to check for outstanding account balances. File away patient charts.
8. Make sure premedicated patients have their medication.
9. Ensure that all lab cases will be delivered before the patient arrives.

10. Type all correspondence as required.
11. Follow up on patients who need to come for a hygiene appointment, patients who have failed appointments or those who need to reschedule.
12. Screen all incoming calls for staff members for call back during their lunch break.
13. Balance the day's receipts with checks, cash, credit card remittances and prepare bank deposit.
14. Make sure that the desk is clean and all charts are put away before leaving for the evening.
15. Smile and communicate with patients in a friendly manner.

Weekly Responsibilities
1. Follow up on all late accounts with a telephone call.
2. Follow up with patients once predeterminations have been received.
3. Reactivate patient charts as time permits.

Monthly Responsibilities
1. Meet with dentist to review the month's production, collections and finances.
2. Write checks for outstanding accounts payable.
3. Attend our monthly staff meeting.

Yearly Responsibilities
1. Meet with dentist for staff evaluation.
2. Meet with dentist for yearly salary review.
3. Attend continuing education seminars/conventions as required.

Team Responsibilities
1. Help to keep the office clean and tidy. Although we have a cleaning company come in each evening, everyone on the team is responsible for the general neatness of their own areas.
2. If time permits, please ask other team members if they require assistance.

Qualities of Our Dental Receptionist
1. Friendly and professional in all dealings with patients.
2. Fair and understanding.
3. The ability to keep patient and practice matters confidential.

4. The ability to remain neutral.
5. Honesty and integrity.
6. Assertiveness.
7. Organizational skills.

THE INTERVIEW

There is no need to have your applicant fill out a job application form, since you have already reviewed their qualifications from the resume and cover letter. However, this is individual to each dental practice.

Ask open-ended questions because you want the applicant to talk about themselves, their qualifications and previous experiences. Try not to ask "yes" or "no" questions. Remember that the applicant is nervous and you may try to put them at ease by offering them juice or coffee.

Prospective employees will also have questions about your dental practice. Not only are you interviewing, but you are also being evaluated by the applicant. Questions by applicants will include some or all of the following:
- initial probation period
- orientation period
- salaries and raises
- work hours and patient hours
- benefits
- holidays
- vacation periods
- sick days, etc.

QUESTIONS TO ASK AT THE INTERVIEW
1. Tell me about your last position. Please outline the duties.
2. How much experience do you have in dentistry?
3. Did you implement any new ideas, systems, programs at your last job? If so, please tell me about them.
4. Why do you feel you are suited to the position available in this practice?
5. Why did you leave your last position?
6. Tell me about your strengths in dentistry. Do you feel there are any areas upon which you need to improve?
7. What do you enjoy most about dentistry?

8. Tell me about your hobbies or interests.

9. How do you feel about continuing education?

10. Are you flexible about working evenings or Saturdays?

11. Would you be willing to work one trial day before we make a final decision?

12. What kind of courses/seminars have you taken in the past?

13. Can I answer any questions for you about the position and our practice?

14. Which previous employer could we call for a reference?

15. How do you feel about talking on the telephone?

16. Do you think you have good communication skills?

17. What are your long-term goals?

A key fact to remember is that there are certain questions you cannot by law ask. Refrain from asking about marriage plans, what their spouse does for a living, do they have children, are they planning on having children, their religion, etc. These types of questions may be a violation of the Human Rights Commission rules. It is important to remember that although many of the applicants may have small children, there is no reason why this would affect their job performance – especially if you have set office hours. If you have informed the applicant of the position's working hours and the amount of flexibility required for the position and they have agreed upon the hours and terms, then there is no need to go beyond that point. Call your provincial/state Human Rights Commission and/or Employment Standards office for their booklet concerning applications, interviews and legally acceptable questions.

When the interview has been completed, remember to thank the applicant for coming in and let them know that you will call them with your decision as soon as possible.

When the applicant has left the office, an interview checklist and comments form should be completed in order to help you remember each applicant's qualities and characteristics. Please see figure 1.1 for a sample Interviewer's Checklist.

THE REFERENCE CHECK

The reference check is an important part of the interview process. It will give you an indication of the applicant's work habits and industriousness. Speak with

FIGURE 1.1   SAMPLE: INTERVIEWER'S CHECKLIST

☐1st Interview   ☐2nd Interview

Applicant's Name: _____
Address   _____
                   _____
Telephone: _____
Position Applied For: _____

	Poor	Satisfactory	Good	Outstanding
Communication Skills	☐	☐	☐	☐
Grammar	☐	☐	☐	☐
Listening Skills	☐	☐	☐	☐
Confidence	☐	☐	☐	☐
Eye Contact	☐	☐	☐	☐
Knowledge of Dentistry	☐	☐	☐	☐
Qualified for Position	☐	☐	☐	☐
Education in Dentistry	☐	☐	☐	☐
Experience	☐	☐	☐	☐
Relevant Questions	☐	☐	☐	☐
Professional Appearance	☐	☐	☐	☐
Attitude/Personality	☐	☐	☐	☐

Total years exp:_____ GP Perio Ortho Endo Prostho Paedo Oral Surgery

Credentials: _____
(Certificates/Degrees):   _____
Supervisory Exp: _____
How Many People: _____
Salary Expectations: _____
Additional Comments: _____
Information Volunteered by Applicant: _____
Reference Check: ☐ Yes ☐ No   _____
Date: _____

the applicant's immediate supervisor as they will have first-hand knowledge of the applicant's skills and qualifications.

Don't rely on only one reference call. I have met wonderful, hardworking people who experienced a personality conflict in previous practices through no fault of their own. These individuals had a negative reference from that practice, but other references turned out to be wonderful. If possible, three reference checks should be made to give you a proper indication of the employee's job performance and attitude. Please see figure 1.2 for a sample Reference Check Form.

FIGURE 1.2   SAMPLE: REFERENCE CHECK FORM

REFERENCE CHECK SHEET

Applicant's Name:
Date:
Dentist's Name:
Reference Name:
Phone:

Nature of work:
Length of time employed:
Reason for leaving:
Attitude towards patients:
Attitude towards co-workers:
Was the applicant industrious:
Outline of duties:

Would you re-hire?:
Would you recommend?:
Strengths:

Weaknesses

Clinical Skills
Additional Comments?

NEGOTIATING SALARIES

DENTAL ASSISTANTS AND RECEPTIONISTS

Each province and state has different wage guidelines for dental team members. The most important thing to remember about salaries is that if you pay low wages, your employees won't be as productive and they will probably be seeking work elsewhere. This doesn't mean that you must pay high wages, only that you pay according to experience and within your practice salary budget (if you have one). Call your local assistants association for the average hourly wage of assistants and receptionists in your geographical area.

All new employees should be on a probationary period for three months in order to determine if they are fully suited to the position. During this time, they should be working on a probationary wage. This means that their pay is slightly less than what you would normally pay. Once the new employee's three-month trial period is over and they have proven their abilities, an increase to regular salary should commence. For example: You hire a dental assistant with two years experience. The regular pay would be $12 per hour but he/she will be paid $11 per hour until the probationary period is over and you are satisfied with the work.

All applicants for positions are usually interested in the rate of pay. At the interview, inform the new applicant of your probationary period, rate of pay during probation and the increase that will be awarded if they are hired permanently. Never pay more than you normally would until you are sure about your new employee.

DENTAL HYGIENISTS
Dental hygienists can be paid in one of three ways.
1. An hourly rate of pay or per day salary.
2. Commission.
3. A combination of per day salary and commission.

By far, the easiest way of compensating dental hygienists is by an hourly rate of pay. This differs from province to province and state to state. Call your hygienist association for average salaries of dental hygienists in your geographical area. If you pay hourly, your practice takes care of all the employment taxes, unemployment insurance, government pensions and income taxes. Although this increases the amount you pay to the government monthly (for payroll taxes), you will have less opportunity for misunderstandings about commissions and contracts. In addition, the hygienist does not have to worry about paying tax in a bulk sum at tax time.

Hygiene contracts are more complicated and more work for both the employer and the employee. It is not necessary to have a contract for each hygienist who works in your practice – unless it is required in your locale. Most hygienists are paid like everyone else in the practice – by an hourly wage or a weekly salary. However, some dentists and hygienists prefer to deal on a contractual basis for a specified period of time. If you pay your hygienists on a commission basis or a base salary plus commission, there must be a signed contract between you to eliminate misunderstandings about billing procedures and frustrations. See the following guidelines for hygiene contracts.

CONTRACT GUIDELINES FOR HYGIENISTS

1. Date of the contract and a future date to review the contract. Contracts for hygienists are usually valid for one year (unless the employment is to cover a sick leave or maternity leave).
2. Hours and days of work must be specified. It should also be noted that the hours are subject to change by the employer with a defined time period of notice.
3. Method of payment (the dentist chooses one).

A. Fixed Salary

The salary is stated in yearly terms (e.g., $35,000 per year) and divided into equal payments depending upon your payroll schedule. For instance, you will be paying your contracted hygienist a salary of $35,000 per year. Your payroll is bi-weekly (26 times per year). The hygienist's rate of pay would be $35,000 divided by 26 paychecks per year or $1346.15.

B. Hourly Pay

Hourly pay is paid for each hour (or fraction of an hour) the dental hygienist is working in the practice. The contract should state the number of hours the hygienist is guaranteed on a per week basis and the payroll schedule (e.g., weekly, bi-weekly, monthly, etc.).

C. Per Diem

Under a per diem salary, the hygienist is paid for each day (or fraction of a day) worked. The contract should state the number of days which the hygienist will work per week and the daily amount (e.g., $220/day for 3.5 days per week). Your payroll schedule should be included as well (weekly, bi-weekly, etc.).

D. Commission Per Patient

A commission per patient is based on the percentage given to the hygienist for each patient's billing (usually 30 to 40%). With the commission contract, there is no base salary. The commission is usually calculated and paid on a monthly basis. The payments could be split according to your payroll schedule (weekly, bi-weekly, etc.).

You must state in the contract the duties and treatment for which commission will be granted and those procedures for which it will not. For example, procedures for which a hygienist should receive commission include:

- Scaling
- Prophylaxis
- Oral hygiene instruction
- Fluoride treatments
- Periodontal evaluations, treatment and charting
- Sealants
- Polishing fillings

Items not covered by commission include:

- Recall examinations
- Incorrect codes/amounts on insurance forms
- Dental x-rays
- Sterilization and other miscellaneous duties which are a part of dental office procedures.
- Any write-off of a billing previously granted as commissionable.

This is by no means a complete list. It is individual to each dentist as to which services will pay a commission to the contracted dental hygienist.

E. Commission Plus Base Salary

This is usually calculated as a base salary per year divided and payable according to your practice's payroll schedule. In addition, a percentage of the gross billings is paid to the hygienist on a monthly basis (or according to the payroll schedule of your practice). As noted previously in this chapter, there are normally certain procedures for which the hygienist is not paid.

F. Self-Employed Hygienists

The self-employed hygienist works much like a contracted hygienist with some exceptions. They are responsible for their own payroll deductions, they are not entitled to staff benefits, nor are they paid for statutory holidays. There is no holiday pay or vacation pay. The self-employed hygienist is usually paid an hourly or per diem rate and signs a contract to work for a specified period in each particular practice.

You should supply the instruments and other items necessary for self-employed hygienists although some will have their own. Self-employed hygienists should be responsible for cleaning and sterilizing their own instruments and treatment room, unless you have an assistant who is responsible for these functions. This should be stated somewhere in the contract in order to eliminate misunderstandings.

4. Other duties the hygienist is to complete should be listed – for instance, sterilization of instruments, calling patients who are due for an appointment, cleaning their area. This section should really be a complete job description of daily, weekly, monthly and team duties.

5. It should be noted that the hygienist must adhere to the rules of the dental practice and to the state/provincial licensing rules of dental hygienists in your area.

6. An overtime policy should be included for all hygienists unless self-employed.

7. Vacation policies and holiday pay should be documented clearly. You should also include any statutory holidays the contracted hygienist is entitled to. Self-employed hygienists are not entitled to holiday pay, although their contract should cover holiday/vacation times.

8. Sick days and procedures must be covered according to practice policy. Self-employed hygienists are not entitled to pay for sick days.

9. Staff benefits should be included. It should be noted that staff benefits are subject to change without notice. Self-employed hygienists are not entitled to benefits.

10. Termination policies must be stated for contracted hygienists. Usually a thirty (30) day written notice of contract termination by either the dentist or the hygienist will suffice. Please refer to your local employment standards office for proper procedures regarding termination.

11. If the contract is violated by either the dentist or the hygienist (or either loses a license to practice), the contract becomes null and void upon notice to the applicable party. Neither the dentist nor the hygienist will be under further obligation, with the exception that the hygienist is entitled to compensation according to the proper employment standards policy of your area.

The contract is then signed and dated by each party. Two copies of the contract are necessary – one for the hygienist and one for the dentist. Please remember that you must take and submit payroll deductions for all contracted hygienists. The only exception are self-employed hygienists, who take care of submitting their own payroll deductions.

THE TRIAL DAY

By far, the best way to determine an applicant's capabilities is to have them come in for one trial day. This will give you an indication of how they function as a team member, with your patients and as a clinical or business auxiliary. The trial day will also show whether the applicant is industrious and takes the initiative to ask questions and learn.

TIPS FOR TRIAL DAYS
1. Schedule trial days on your least busy day so that you will have a better chance to observe the applicant.
2. All applicants should be paid for trial days even if they volunteer to work for free.
3. Appoint a helper for your applicant. This person will spend the day with them, showing them around, giving them a feel for office policies and procedures.
4. Make notes about your applicant for later referral. Use a checklist and mark off duties they can do and the ones that will require further training. This will help to make your decision easier.
5. Compliment your applicant. Praise will boost their self-confidence.
6. Remember, the new applicant will be nervous. Keep this in mind when observing how they work.

PROBATIONARY PERIOD

Once you have made your decision to hire a new employee, you must set a trial period. This can range anywhere from two weeks to three months. An average probationary period is usually three months. This will give you and your team members more than enough time to determine whether the new employee is truly the right person for the job – within a couple of weeks you will know whether the person is going to work out. You will see how they fit in with your existing team members and how they interact with patients. During the probationary period, the new employee should be considered a temporary whose permanent employment with your practice is pending.

At the end of the trial period, if not before, a meeting should be set up between you and the new employee to discuss permanent employment, salary, benefits and evaluations. At this point, if hired, the employee should be given a raise to the regular rate of pay. If you notice within a couple of weeks that the employee will not work out in your practice, let them go. Don't suffer through three months when you can use the time to find someone who is suitable.

"The only companies that grow are the ones that expect their people to grow and spend the time and money to do it."

William Marsteller

ORIENTATION PERIOD

The orientation period coincides with the probation period. This is often a trying time for your new employee, who will be nervous about fitting in and completing tasks accurately and on time. This is also a time of frustration for the dentist, who must cope with training and orienting the new employee. A few simple guidelines can help to ease your new team member into their position.

1. Set aside training time. Setting aside time to train your new team member is essential. Each and every office is unique and therefore a period of adjustment will be necessary. Depending upon the job responsibilities and previous experience of the employee, training times will differ for each person. Keep in mind that even if the person has 20 years of assisting experience, training is still necessary to help the person adjust to your office procedures.

2. Offer personal support. Praise and compliment your new team member when they are doing something right. Supporting people raises their self-confidence and makes them want to try harder.

3. Offer constructive comments. If your employee is having trouble with a

certain procedure, show them an easier way of doing it and offer more training if it is required.

4. Involve other team members. Everyone should try to help the new employee adjust. Share the responsibility, as a dental practice should be a team environment.

5. Communicate your expectations. The new team member must have a clear understanding of what is expected of them. Provide them with a detailed job description.

Most important, don't procrastinate if the new employee is not working out. If you have provided ample training, support and expectations and the employee has not responded, let them go. The longer you keep an inappropriate applicant, the harder it will be to terminate their employment.

SALARY AND BENEFIT GUIDES

All new applicants are interested in salary and benefits. These subjects should be generally covered at the interview. Once you have made your decision and start your employee on probation, a salary and benefit guide should be filled out to eliminate misunderstandings about pay, trial periods, evaluations, etc. Please see figure 1.3 for a sample Salary and Benefit Guide. This form should be filled out in duplicate: one copy for office/payroll records and one copy to be retained by the employee.

STAFF EVALUATIONS

All employees should have a staff evaluation at least once per year. The purpose of the evaluation is to help your employees to improve their job performance. Evaluations are conducted:
1. At the end of the probationary period.
2. For all employees on an annual basis.
3. For disciplinary reviews.

FIGURE 1.3   SAMPLE: SALARY AND BENEFIT GUIDE

EMPLOYER: _____   **EMPLOYEE:** _____

POSITION: _____   **DATE OF EMPLOYMENT:** _____
S. I. N. (or SS#): _____
PREPARED BY: _____   **DATE:** _____

Probationary Rate of Pay: _____   Increasing to _____
(For three months)
Total Annual Salary: _____   Hourly Rate _____
Total Hours/Day _____   Hours/Week: _____

Date of Trial Period Review _____
(3 months for new employees)
Date of Staff Evaluation: _____
(One per year for employees)
Salary Review Date: _____
(usually 3 months for new employees/one
per year for all employees)

BENEFITS
Incentive Bonus:
Uniform Allowance _____
Dental Benefits: _____
Life Insurance/Prescriptions _____
Medical Insurance: _____

SICK/WELLNESS DAYS
Total number paid sick days/year _____
Personal/Wellness days (if applicable) _____

OTHER BENEFITS
Continuing education days per year: _____
Paid conventions and/or seminars _____
Professional Dues: _____

VACATION/HOLIDAYS
Total number statutory holidays
employee will be paid for per year _____
Vacation Pay: _____
When can vacation be taken _____

Employer's Signature: _____   **Employee's Signature:** _____

Evaluations help you to help your team. They should include a written account of the team member's strengths and weaknesses, areas of improvement, progress and salary increase (if applicable).

Yearly evaluations should be conducted privately between the dentist and employee or between an office administrator and the employee. The results of evaluations should be kept confidential from other team members. See figure 1.4 for a sample Staff Evaluation Form.

HIRING AN ASSOCIATE DENTIST

If you have a very busy practice and patients are unable to get an appointment for weeks in advance, it is time to think of hiring an associate dentist. Or perhaps you wish to increase the productivity of your practice or you want to work fewer hours. An associate dentist can help with all of these areas.

Many dentists hire an associate a few years before they are ready to retire, with plans of selling the practice to the new associate. Others hire associates because the practice has become too busy for one dentist to handle. In either case, the associate must be compatible with your practice and patient philosophies.

Before hiring an associate, make sure that you have fully considered the following possibilities:

1. How much can the practice pay an associate?
2. Will you pay them a salary, base salary plus commission or strictly commission?
3. Do you have enough work to accommodate an associate?
4. Will you have to hire other staff to work with the associate?
5. Are you hiring an associate with the intention of having them purchase the practice?
6. If so, what is the value of the practice?
7. When will the associate be able to purchase the practice?
8. What will be the cost of the buy-in?
9. How will the buy-in be completed?
10. Do you have the necessary room for an associate?

(NOTE: For details on practice valuations and buy-in contracts, it is recommended that you contact a local broker and lawyer who are experienced in these matters.)

FIGURE 1.4   SAMPLE: STANDARD STAFF EVALUATION FORM

Employee Name		Position	
Date of Employment		Date of Review	
Beginning Salary	Present Salary	Amount of Last Raise/Date	Proposed Increase/Effective Date

Purpose of Review   ❏Completion of trial period   ❏Annual Salary Review   ❏Disciplinary Review

	POOR	FAIR	SATISFACTORY	GOOD	EXCELLENT
Punctuality	❏	❏	❏	❏	❏
Attendance	❏	❏	❏	❏	❏
Dependability	❏	❏	❏	❏	❏
Initiative/Motivation	❏	❏	❏	❏	❏
Knowledge of position	❏	❏	❏	❏	❏
Ability to learn new techniques	❏	❏	❏	❏	❏
Judgement - Makes sound decisions	❏	❏	❏	❏	❏
Cooperation with others	❏	❏	❏	❏	❏
Attitude in the practice	❏	❏	❏	❏	❏
Attitude with patients	❏	❏	❏	❏	❏
Quality of work/accuracy	❏	❏	❏	❏	❏
Speed - Rate of work	❏	❏	❏	❏	❏

EMPLOYEE'S STRENGTHS	EMPLOYEE'S WEAKNESSES

Since the last raise this employee has: ❏Made progress   ❏Made no changes   ❏Regressed

COMMENTS

_____
_____
_____
_____
_____
_____
_____
_____
_____

Recommended Salary Increase   ❏YES   ❏No   Amount:

Signature of Employer: _____

Signature of Employee: _____

Once you have answered these questions (and documented them for later referral) you can begin to look for an associate. Hiring an associate is much like hiring a staff member. You are looking for someone with the right qualities, attitude, experience and work habits, who will fit into your practice and be compatible with the rest of your team. As noted previously in this chapter, make out a list of the qualities and experience you are looking for in an associate. This is even more important if you are hiring the associate with the intent of having them purchase your practice when you retire. You want your patients to receive the same type of care and service they received from you.

PLACES TO FIND AN ASSOCIATE
- Dental school journals. If you are willing to take on an inexperienced dentist who will require training, your best source will be a dental school. Most have journals where you can place a classified advertisement.
- Dental journals and publications. Most provincial/state associations have a section for classified advertisements. Many dentists hire their associates this way. The national dental journals provide a suitable way to advertise as well. Many associates are willing to relocate for a good, solid position in a dental practice – especially if they will have the option to buy into the practice in future years.
- Newspaper classifieds are also a great way to advertise. This is usually more successful in major cities with a large population base from which to receive applicants.
- Word-of-mouth referrals.

A written contract is critical for associate dentists. Never hire an associate dentist over a handshake. You must have a written contract to avoid misunderstandings and disputes. It is highly recommended that you have your lawyer review the contract before either party signs the agreement.

LOCUMS

Often dentists postpone their vacations due to revenue loss while they must still carry overhead costs. To combat part of this problem, the dentist should have the team take part of their vacation while the dentist is on vacation (which should be stated in your office policy manual). If your hygienists are legally able to work independently (depending on the laws in your state, province or country), this will help the practice's productivity, but in many locations hygienists are required to have a dentist in the office while they have patients scheduled. The answer is to hire a locum while you take a vacation.

HOW DO YOU FIND A LOCUM?
- Word of mouth.
- Advertise in dental journals.
- Call local dental associations.
- Call universities for names of recent graduates.

New graduates may be slower and somewhat inexperienced but they can work with your hygiene team and look after any emergency patients while you are away.

As with any potential employee, always make sure that you check several references to ensure that you are comfortable that the locum will take excellent care of your patients. Please refer to figure 1.2 for a sample of Reference Check Questions to ask. Other questions of importance include:
- How did the locum dentist relate to your patients?
- Was your team comfortable with him/her?
- Were you pleased with the quality of dentistry?
- Were your patients happy?

Hiring a locum is not for everyone, but it is an option that is worth looking into.

SUMMARY
- Take the time to review staffing needs.
- What personality type do you feel would complement your practice?
- Have a detailed list of requirements needed for the available position.
- List the type of experience required.
- Be realistic regarding the training time that will be involved.
- List your team requirements and discuss potential applicants with them.
- Plan uninterrupted interview time.
- Coordinate observation time in the practice.
- Make a decision.
- Have a set probationary period for your new team member.
- EVALUATE, TRAIN & COMMUNICATE.

AREAS OUR PRACTICE CAN IMPROVE UPON

NOTES

"The first step toward success in any job is to become interested in it."
William Osler

2.

LEADERSHIP SKILLS

"The task of the leader is to get his people from where they are to where they have not been."

Henry Kissinger

FIVE TYPES OF DENTISTS

1. MR. NICE GUY

This dentist is too nice. He lets his staff do what they want and in far too many cases, the staff dictates to the dentist about the running of the practice – often in front of patients. This dentist eventually loses control of the practice and staff to a more dominant personality. With the loss of control comes the loss of respect.

2. THE DICTATOR

"*My* way or the highway" is the message from this dentist. This dentist does not listen to his staff and feels he has all the answers. If staff don't like it, they can be replaced. This dentist has a high staff turnover in the practice and lower than average new patient numbers. The staff who work in this practice are not part of a team and to them, their position is often "just a job".

3. INCONSISTENT DENTISTS

Some days he is Mr. Nice Guy and some days he is the Dictator. Often this type of doctor will have set policies and guidelines for staff and patients but won't enforce them until under duress. This dentist easily loses the respect of his team through his inconsistencies.

4. **Mr. Friendly**

The practice is more of a social gathering where everyone is the best of friends and do not take the business side of dentistry as seriously as it should be taken. Being friendly is great, but there is a fine line you cannot cross if you are the employer. In this type of practice, patients and staff enjoy the friendly atmosphere but don't take financial commitments or discipline seriously. This dentist generally has financial problems and is unable to control expenditures.

5. **Leaders by Example**

Dentists who lead by example are often enthusiastic about their practice, communicate with their staff and hold regular meetings. The staff have defined duties and the dentist's expectations are shared with staff. This dentist often sets practice goals and shares them with the team. His practice is progressive and productive. To become a leader by example takes time and discipline but it is truly the only way to a successful and harmonious dental practice.

When you change your attitude and begin to lead by example, the people around you will respond in a similar manner. Enthusiasm and motivation bring out the best in people. Staff will take the initiative, be more productive and most important, they will be happy. A happy staff is a productive staff and patients tend to refer to happy, productive practices.

Saying No and Staying Neutral

It is difficult for some dentists to say "no" as it is difficult for some dentists to listen to their staff. That's okay because no one is perfect. This is why we promote teamwork and shared leadership. The dentist is the one who should set the policies and guidelines for the staff to follow and enforce. An office coordinator or administrator can enforce the policies of the practice in an assertive but professional way. Disputes and disagreements – if not sorted out by the team – are brought to the attention of the dentist. As the business owner and employer, the dentist should have the final word on policy.

It takes a special person to listen attentively and to stay neutral in staff or patient disputes. However, with set policies and guidelines, the dentist can eliminate some of the stress and frustration by remaining neutral and referring to the consistent policies that are in place.

TIPS FOR SAYING NO AND REMAINING NEUTRAL

- Encourage the entire team to help set office policies and ensure that everyone has agreed to the policies.
- As the leader, you must enforce the policies you set.
- Encourage all staff members to work out problems with each other before coming to you.
- Don't let anyone manipulate you or try to corner you.
- Know and be very clear about your reasons for saying no.
- Appoint an office administrator to deal with the day-to-day running of the practice and personnel responsibilities.
- Encourage open communication in your office.
- Be a positive role model for your team. If you are always positive and energetic, chances are, your staff will try to follow in your footsteps.
- Be fair but don't let anyone take advantage of you.

BALANCING FAMILY AND LEISURE TIME WITH WORK

Some dentists find it difficult to balance family and work, often spending evenings or weekends in the practice. The dentists who have outside interests and set practice hours appear happier and more content during their practice hours. Plan how many clinical hours you are comfortable working, allow time for administration and write your hours down. Over the years, I have noticed that dentists can be more efficient and productive with condensed clinical hours rather than spreading their work over five or six days.

If possible, schedule vacation time well in advance. Don't keep working, telling yourself you are too solidly booked and don't have time for a vacation. Keep in mind that for single producers the production stops unless they are in area which permits hygienists to see patients while the doctor is absent. To combat this fear, hire a locum to generate income while you are away. For those who do not want to hire a locum, a good financial budget can account for time off for vacations.

Continuing education seminars in different locations can serve as business/ personal vacations. Many conventions cater to spouses and children as well as dentists. Mental health days allow you to return to the office refreshed, relaxed and motivated.

It is important to the team that during clinical time, a dentist limits personal phone calls and/or social planning which interrupt an otherwise well scheduled day. Interruptions keep patients waiting. If you have other matters to deal with, try to plan your telephone time around your clinical hours.

TIPS FOR BALANCING FAMILY AND LEISURE TIME
- Planned, organized workdays are much less stressful than scattered hours.
- Working longer hours does not guarantee success.
- Make sure that you take time off each year for a vacation with family and friends.
- Take a couple of mental health days off each year. These can be planned in advance. Remember that taking two days off each year is not going to make or break your practice.
- Reduce your evening and weekend hours to spend time with family and friends. Alternate Saturdays and one or two evenings per week are more than sufficient for most dental practices – depending on your location.

HOW TO GET THE BEST FROM YOUR TEAM

"It is not the mountain we conquer, but ourselves."
Sir Edmund Hillary

Your team is only as motivated and enthusiastic as you. Encourage staff members to grow in their positions by delegating duties to trained team members. This increases their self-esteem and motivation. If you take time to listen to your team's ideas and goals, you will learn more about them as individuals.

If there is someone on your team who isn't interested or who is negative, ask yourself if this person complements the practice or are they a liability? If they are uninterested in you and the practice, how are they with your patients?

TIPS FOR GETTING THE BEST FROM YOUR TEAM
- Hold regular team meetings and encourage ideas from team members.
- Have one-on-one meetings for training, ideas and motivation.
- Be enthusiastic and committed. Leaders lead by example and an enthusiastic leader will have a motivated team.
- Give recognition and appreciation for a job well done. "*Thank you*" is the best motivator of all.

- Always have defined duties for competent staff so that they are aware of their responsibilities.
- Delegate duties to trained and competent staff. More challenge for staff means more self-confidence. More self-confidence promotes productivity and a positive attitude.

MANAGING OFFICE CONFLICTS

"It isn't the people you fire who will make your life miserable, it's the people you don't fire."

Harvey Mackay

In any business there will always be a certain amount of conflict as long as two or more people are working together. It is normal to feel frustrated, concerned, jealous or stressed at times. Even if we like the person we are working with, there will be times when our views or methods of operation conflict. The majority of office conflicts are minor and are usually worked out among the individuals involved. There are times when conflict lingers and tension results among team members. You cannot ignore conflict because patients hear it, see it and feel it.

In the event of a staff conflict, it should be made clear that both parties need to resolve their conflict privately, one-on-one. This should be the first course of action rather than third-party arbitration. We don't have to like everyone we work with but we should recognize their ability and contribution to the practice.

Unfortunately, some people are unable or unwilling to resolve their conflicts. If the argument cannot be resolved, the dentist should give each party a 30-day written warning to correct their behavior, as their attitudes are detrimental to the practice, the staff and the patients. Please see figure 2.1 for a sample Warning Letter to Staff Members.

Lingering conflicts create animosity among staff and reduce the productivity of the team. If one person is a trouble maker, you must ask yourself if you really need the aggravation and the negative behavior in your practice. Why pay someone to make everyone else (including you) unhappy?

TIPS FOR REDUCING OFFICE CONFLICTS
- Encourage open communication in your practice. If staff members are able to voice ideas and suggestions openly for team discussion, a consensus can be reached, thereby avoiding arguments.

FIGURE 2.1   SAMPLE: WARNING LETTER TO STAFF MEMBER

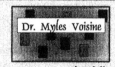

Dr. Myles Voisine

1400-239 East Churchill Road
Harrisford, New Jersey 03040
(409) 555-6114

January 23, 1996
Ms. Sabrina Hadfield

Dear Sabrina,

You are a valuable member of my dental team and I truly appreciate your contribution to the practice. However, your attitude and personal conflict with our other team member, Alana Beck, has become detrimental to our practice.

Conflict lowers office morale and creates a stressful atmosphere for our other team members and our patients. It is important that you make every effort to resolve your conflict with Alana within 30 days. As the practice owner and employer, I am quite willing to arbitrate between you should you be unable to resolve your conflict privately.

Dr. Myles Voisine

NOTE TO DENTISTS: Please check with your local employment standards office for government regulations on written notice and termination of employment. This differs from area to area.

Cosmetic & Restorative Dentistry

- Treat all staff members equally. Favoritism promotes conflict, competition and rumors.
- Put your office policies in writing in a simple office manual. If your policies are firm and consistent, you will limit the climate for conflicts to grow.
- Ensure that all team members have clearly defined responsibilities. There will be overlap in some areas but each team member should know what they are specifically responsible for on a daily basis.
- Listen to your entire team. Don't let one person control your practice.

"An important task of a leader is to reduce his people's excuses for failure."
Robert Townsend

MAINTAINING CONTROL WHILE GIVING THE FREEDOM TO BE EFFECTIVE

Once office policies are clear and each team member has clearly defined duties, let each person know how far they can go using their own initiative. For example, when making financial arrangements, can your receptionist make payment decisions without checking with you first? Your office policy states that payment may be made over a two month period and a patient has requested a three-month payment plan. Does the business assistant have your permission to be flexible and if so, to what extent?

Regular team meetings are important for maintaining control of your practice. Each person should give a report on their area of the practice to discuss concerns, new ideas and completion of regular duties. If the hygiene coordinator hasn't had time to follow up on perio patients who postpone appointments, you need to know why. If there is down-time in your schedule, the appointment secretary needs to know exactly how much this is costing the practice and you both need to discuss ways to solve the down-time problem. The dentist must see the results and listen to staff concerns and then the team should discuss how to be more effective.

Tips for Maintaining Control
- Always communicate with your staff. Make certain they understand your expectations. Listen to their concerns.
- Be clear and consistent with your office policies. Enforce your written policies when necessary – don't back off or you will start to lose control.

- Set team goals. Give everyone on your staff something to work towards.

MUTUAL RESPECT

"I am always ready to learn although I do not always like to be taught."
Winston Churchill

Try to concentrate on the good qualities of each person on your team. Remember that you hired them so you must have had confidence in them at some point. We all need to recognize that no one is perfect, but we all have something to offer as individuals. It is equally important that your team believe in your dentistry. Mutual respect creates a positive environment for patients. The more confidence your patients have in you and your practice, the higher their acceptance of comprehensive care. Listen to the way people speak to each other. You can tell by the tone of voice if there is mutual respect between people.

TIPS FOR BUILDING MUTUAL RESPECT IN THE PRACTICE

- List the good qualities of each team member and let them know how important they are to the success of your practice.
- Make the time for private conversations. Ask team members exactly where they can make improvements to their job performance.
- Be aware of your tone of voice and your body language. There is nothing worse or more demeaning for an assistant than a dentist who rolls his eyes or sighs loudly while she is trying to perform her job. If you belittle people, you belittle yourself.
- Encourage team members who need extra help. If they are positive, enthusiastic and great with patients, help them to be more productive by providing extra training. Loyalty is one of the best qualities in a person.
- Never forget employees who give 150% of themselves to the practice.
- Don't reprimand a staff member in front of others – do it privately.

DECISION MAKING MADE EASY

"Decisions put us in charge of our own lives."
Theodore Isaac Rubin

Many dentists are notorious for procrastinating. Procrastination causes stress because you worry about things which are not done. One of the fastest ways to demotivate an enthusiastic team who are full of new ideas is to say:

- *"Let me think about it."*
- *"We'll see about that in a few months."*
- *"Let me talk to my friends."*

ARE YOU A PROCRASTINATOR?

- Do you end up at the mall on December 24th?
- Do you miss concerts or plays because you never got around to getting tickets?
- Do you have a pile of charts on your desk waiting for treatment plans?
- Do you postpone decorating your office or purchasing a computer?
- Do you tend to put off staff reprimands because you cannot deal with confrontations?

As a business owner you must make decisions in order to move ahead and have your business grow. Planning is important; don't rely on undefined or vague thoughts. Questions to ask regarding your plans and decisions include:

- What results do I want to achieve?
- What will happen if things stay the way they are now?
- What can I delegate to my team?
- Do I have the support I need?
- How long will it take to accomplish my plan/goal?

IDEAS FOR DECISION MAKING

1. Focus on the benefits of the plan.
2. Clarify the obstacles you will need to overcome in order to achieve success.
3. Make sure that you do proper research and gather as much information as you can before making decisions.
4. Include your team's ideas and thoughts in your decision making. You may have a balance of talent (long-range and short-range thinkers along with both creative and practical thinkers).

MEETING METHOD FOR DECISION MAKING

1. Plan a meeting. If the decision affects the entire team, invite them to join you. If the decision is a financial one, you may wish to share it with your team or your office manager. Keep in mind that two heads are better than one and will come up with more ideas and solutions.

2. Have an agenda. This includes setting a method and a deadline date.

3. Be clear about your budget. Don't go overboard thinking that you'll find the extra money somewhere. Set an amount you can afford and stick with it.

4. Encourage communication from everyone involved and listen to all comments objectively.

5. Document all comments from your meeting and distribute the notes within two days. It is best to keep notes rather than try to remember every idea and solution mentioned during a meeting, and by distributing them, all members of the team will have the same understanding of events.

6. Review all of your ideas, solutions and alternatives and then sleep on it. Many managers or business owners need time to absorb and think things over after a meeting, so ensure that you have set yourself a deadline for your decision. Share your decision with your team and then begin work on your project.

PREPARING FOR CHANGE BY BREAKING OLD HABITS

"When you're through changing, you're through."
Bruce Barton

Making a change is the hardest part once you have made a decision – getting the work completed is usually much easier. People fear change – the fear of failure or of rejection. As a good friend of mine admitted, most of us don't change until we feel the pain – until it hurts emotionally, financially or socially. Why wait?

We know the world changes. Look back to dentistry twenty years ago, ten years ago and as recently as five years ago. There have been major changes with products, techniques, infection control, computerization, procedures and dental insurance to name just a few. In five, ten or twenty years, dentistry will continue to evolve. With improved technology, these changes will be happening more rapidly.

To make changes we need to look at our business. What needs to change? How effective are our systems and overall practice? Areas to look at include:

• Collections
• Your attitude
• Accounting procedures
• Insurance

- Recall system
- Periodontal programs
- Scheduling
- Patient follow-up
- Team meetings
- Leadership skills
- Financial control
- Patient education
- Staff education
- Computer system

This list could be endless. Each practice is unique so you really need to ask yourself what could be better. Be specific. It is important to understand that people feel uncomfortable with change and need the support of others. Keep in mind that some people refuse to make changes. If you have people in your practice who resist change, it will hold your practice back. They will eventually demotivate others on your team by saying things such as:

- *"We tried something like that before."*
- *"Things are fine just the way they are now."*
- *"We don't have time for this."*

These people find it easier to do things the way they have always been done. They are afraid to change and in fact may not be able to handle the changes. Support for each other on the team is essential in order for change to occur. You must encourage each other towards the new project. If any team member totally resists changes, you need to ask yourself, *"Do I need all of these negative comments?"* Someone once said, *"It is easier to run with 20 people than with one person tied around your neck."* Support is essential because if you lose your focus, it is very easy to slip back into old habits and systems.

TIPS FOR PREPARING FOR CHANGE

- Make sure that your entire team is aware that you are serious about making changes.
- Include deadlines, details and methods in your plan. Keep in mind that you must allow some flexibility.
- Encourage each other. Making changes is hard and everyone needs encouragement.

- Think of the advantages and benefits your changes will bring to the team and the practice.
- Don't wait too long to change.

COPING WITH STRESS IN THE PRACTICE

At seminars when I ask the audience, *"Is there any stress in dentistry?"* the audience always roars back, *"YES."* On a positive note, we must remember that most of what we worry about never happens.

Stress comes in two forms: negative stress and positive stress. Negative stress is stress that we cannot control such as fires, accidents, getting stuck in elevators or traffic. We deal with negative stress as individuals – usually panic first then relief.

Positive stress is stress that we can control. It gets our adrenaline going. It is important to identify the source of your positive stress and then to come up with solutions to minimize it.

Many times we cause our own stress:
- Running behind schedule.
- Frustrations with incompetent staff.
- Becoming upset when patients don't pay.
- Finding out patients have spent their insurance check.
- Having a patient in the chair and their case is not back from the lab.
- Cash flow has become tight or inadequate.

There are practical solutions to eliminate such problems. Stress is caused by not having a practice plan, by failing to enforce policies, and by burying our heads in the sand and hoping it all goes away. It is important that we deal with stress or it can cause problems such as eating disorders, insomnia, heart attacks, burnout, not enjoying each work day, etc.

As in all cases such as decision making or practice planning, the number one thing to do is to identify the source of your stress.

1. What is causing your stress?
2. How can you eliminate the stress?
3. What obstacles do you need to overcome?
4. How will you feel when the stress has been eliminated?
5. How will you feel if you continue to ignore the problem which is causing you stress?

Make it happen; each day is special. Enjoy it and get rid of the clutter in your life.

"If it is not life threatening, don't worry about it."
Dr. Peter Clark

ORGANIZATIONAL SKILLS – CONTROL OF SYSTEMS

There is far too much lost revenue in dentistry due to poorly organized systems and a lack of follow-up. Often in practices, I see too many people doing the same thing. Each individual must be accountable for their own duties.

Review each system in your practice (recall, insurance, financial, scheduling, inventory).

- How organized is it? Can you find the information you need quickly? Can you make easy referral to your system?
- How effective is it? Do patients or payments slip through the cracks?
- How do you follow up? Is someone responsible for following up? How efficient is the follow-up?
- Do you have the right staff for the job? Are they positive? Productive? Do they really know what they are doing? Have you trained them properly?
- How efficient is your lab? Do you receive your cases on time?
- On your own desk, do you have piles of charts all over the place? Can you actually see your desk? Can you find what you are looking for when you need it?
- Is your personal and office filing system organized? Is it easy to pull charts? Do you misplace charts on a regular basis? Is there some type of order to your filing system? Are files labeled? Are files color-coded? Do you play that game, "Let's hunt for the patient chart?"

TIPS FOR STAYING ORGANIZED
- Only keep files on your desk which need to be dealt with immediately.
- Open up "To Do" files for the week and for the month. Make sure that each file is cleared by your weekly or monthly deadline.
- Get rid of junk – old books, old papers, etc.
- Have an "In" file for daily review (such as mail, incoming letters, etc.).
- Have an "Out" file for things to be mailed or delegated to a competent assistant or business assistant.
- Set aside 2 to 4 hours per week (without patients) for organizational time

to clear your desk and your files and to catch up on paperwork.
- Use a daily priority list (see figure 2.2). List the people to call for the day and the paperwork priorities you need to deal with.

We all have our own way of doing things but the more organized you are with your business systems, the more productive you will be with your time.

Plan organizational time for your practice and your team on a monthly or bi-monthly basis. Set aside half a day or a full day for everyone on the team to catch up, file and sort. Make and keep the commitment to be organized.

KEEPING UP TO DATE WITH CHANGES IN DENTISTRY

Patients want to know that you and your team are using the most up-to-date techniques and equipment. They want to know that you are an excellent dentist. A patient's greatest fear is still *pain*. Let patients know that by keeping up to date with technology, your practice can provide a comfortable dental experience.

Often dentists take courses but don't share the information with the team, who have no idea what is happening when the dentist uses a new technique on a patient. When dentists take courses or seminars, the following points should be remembered so that the entire team can benefit from your newly gained knowledge:

1. Plan a one-hour staff meeting within three days of the course.
2. Share the information you have learned.
3. Train the staff about the new techniques.
4. Discuss with everyone how you can introduce it into your practice.
5. List the advantages to the patient and the practice.
6. Sort out and discuss insurance coverage and treatment fees.
7. Discuss how to schedule.
8. Discuss staff training (if required).

If you do not educate your staff, they will have no idea what is happening. If a patient asks them questions about the new procedure, they will have to answer, "I don't know". You want your staff to be knowledgeable and up to date because it will benefit your practice and the team. Take the time to share your new knowledge with them. There are far too many new procedures, products or techniques that are never used because there has been no follow-through.

FIGURE 2.2   SAMPLE: DAILY PRIORITY LIST

Things to Do On:_____

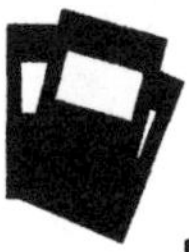

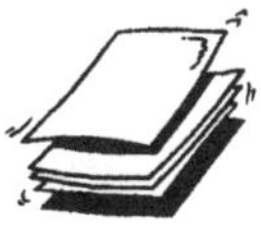

Tasks To Complete   ### Daily Schedule

☑ check when completed

Tasks	Daily Schedule
❑ _____	6:00 AM
❑ _____	7:00
❑ _____	8:00
❑ _____	9:00
❑ _____	10:00
❑ _____	11:00
❑ _____	12:00 PM
❑ _____	1:00
❑ _____	2:00
❑ _____	3:00
❑ _____	4:00
❑ _____	5:00
❑ _____	6:00
❑ _____	7:00
❑ _____	8:00
❑ _____	9:00
❑ _____	10:00
❑ _____	11:00
❑ _____	12:00 AM

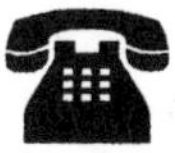

Telephone Calls to Make

❑ _____   _____
❑ _____   _____
❑ _____   _____
❑ _____   _____
❑ _____   _____
❑ _____   _____
❑ _____   _____

Some practices are using computers which are outdated, overloaded, slow and inefficient. It is important to update both your hardware and software. Fast, efficient equipment is worth its weight in gold. The same goes for intraoral cameras. I have seen so many practices with cameras which just sit there and collect dust instead of being used as a powerful patient education tool for practice building.

If you have new equipment and services:
- Train your team.
- Decide who can use the technique and equipment.
- Let your patients know about the new services and procedures available.
- Educate your patients.

SETTING PRACTICE GOALS

Most dentists (and others) do not set goals. They may think about them and have vague ideas, but the majority do not write them down and formulate plans to achieve those goals. People who take the time to write down their goals and their visions are usually the ones to reach those goals and ultimately build an even more successful business.

Goals to think about (on a one-year, five-year and ten-year basis) include:
1. Educational goals (all staff).
2. Career goals.
3. Production goals.
4. New patient numbers.
5. Collection goals.
6. Marketing goals.
7. Retirement goals.

TIPS FOR GOAL SETTING
- Be realistic. Don't set your next monthly production goal at $35,000 if your average monthly production is usually $25,000. Try for a $2000 or $2500 increase rather than $10,000. By setting goals too high, you demotivate yourself and your team when the goal is not reached.
- Be specific. Instead of saying, "This month I'm going to increase my new patient numbers," say instead, "This month my goal to achieve is 35 new patients".
- Review your goals on a monthly basis in order to stay on track. Reviewing goals also serves as a basis for motivation and enthusiasm.

• Share your goals with your team. They cannot help you if they don't know what you want to achieve.

MANAGING YOUR TIME

"Waste neither time nor money, but make the best of both."
Benjamin Franklin

Once you get organized with your practice systems, you need to manage your time properly. I rarely run out of energy, but I often run out of time. The main way to organize your time is to prioritize it. This is what I have become an expert at, travelling the way I do.

1. Set your clinical hours and have separate time for phone calls, business planning and meetings.
2. Work from a Daily Priority List. See the sample in this chapter (figure 2.2).
3. Always highlight the urgent and difficult things to do first and get them out of your way. It is far too easy to do the simple and little things first – which is what most people do.
4. Don't interrupt your clinical time with phone calls and other duties or you will fall behind schedule and cause stress for yourself, your staff and your patients.

They always say if you want something done, ask a busy person. Many people spend only 25% of their time on important things and the rest on bits and pieces. Reverse this trend and you will be able to control your time more effectively. One of the main problems is that many dentists try to do too much themselves. Delegation to competent staff can help. Allow your team to make decisions in order to eliminate the many daily interruptions.

Most of all, you need quiet, uninterrupted time to focus on your priorities. Time needs to be divided into:

• Family and social time.
• Personal leisure time for hobbies, sports, etc.
• Clinical time.
• Business, administration, organizational, educational time.

Work out the percentage for each category to meet your personal needs – then relax and enjoy.

STAFF TRAINING AND DELEGATION OF DUTIES

Delegation gives your dental team the opportunity to grow personally and professionally. It offers them challenge and self-confidence. Delegation offers you the chance to delete some duties from your busy schedule. It does not mean that you are allowing your team to make decisions and run the practice. You still retain control but have provided your team with the freedom to be more effective.

Listen to all staff suggestions and remember that the final decision will always be yours.

TASKS WHICH COULD BE DELEGATED TO TRAINED TEAM MEMBERS:
(other than regular duties)
- Opening and sorting mail.
- Accounts Payable.
- Patient education.
- Intraoral camera.
- Reinforcing treatment plans.
- Leading staff meetings.

Training time should be set aside before you delegate duties. There is not much point in delegating to a staff member who doesn't know what they are doing. It is important to actually schedule time in the appointment book for staff training. Set an agenda for staff training and ask your staff:
- What would they like to do more of if they could?
- What are they good at?
- What other responsibilities would they like to assume?
- Where do they require/desire more training?
- How could they improve their job performance?

Remember that being unable to delegate can have a negative effect on a practice. The fear of loss of power is the reason why some managers don't delegate.

BUILDING A PROFESSIONAL RELATIONSHIP WITH YOUR TEAM

It is hard to like everyone all of the time. Working together is like a marriage – we spend more time with our associates than with the people we love and live with. Being too friendly and personally involved with each other's personal life is not a great way to begin or end a business relationship. As the dentist, you are the employer. If you become too friendly with your staff, it will become increasingly harder to enforce or implement new policies. There is nothing wrong with being friendly and social with staff; however, it can hold you back from telling your team if they are not meeting your expectations.

There is a fine line between being the friendly boss and being too nice and flexible. The opposite can also happen if the dentist is "The Boss" and staff feel uncomfortable taking concerns or suggestions to the dentist. It is important to understand each other as individuals. This will allow you to identify each other's unique qualities and creativity.

TIPS FOR BUILDING A PROFESSIONAL RELATIONSHIP

- Leave personal problems at home. Don't bring them to work to discuss with your staff. Leave your spouse or mother at home when you come to work. There is nothing wrong with discussing families and spouses, but don't discuss your marriage problems or spouse's personal habits.
- Know each other's qualities and recognize the contribution they make to your practice.
- Save social conversations for lunch or breaks. In front of patients, the talk should concern dentistry or small talk.
- Implement and enforce staff office policies in a consistent manner.
- Lead by example.
- Remember that your patients are your number-one priority – your practice is not a place for social gathering.
- There is life after dentistry.

Building a professional relationship can be accomplished if you have the ability to communicate effectively, to be a team player. Remember that a good sense of humor always helps. Patients love laughter, so laugh with them; there is nothing unprofessional about being happy.

AREAS OUR PRACTICE CAN IMPROVE UPON

NOTES

"Leadership is the ability to hide your panic from others"
Anita Jupp

3.

SETTING OFFICE POLICIES

"Today's preparation determines tomorrow's achievement."
Unknown

SETTING OFFICE POLICIES FOR YOUR MANUAL

Please refer to your province/state employment standards agency before finalizing any policies in your office manual. The following policies should *always* be included in any office policy manual:

- Office hours
- Working hours vs. patient hours
- Staff appearance: jewelry, nail polish, uniforms, shoes, lab coats, etc.
- Job description for each position in the practice
- Staff benefits for full- and part-time employees
- Any incentive bonus plan(s) you may have
- Probationary periods
- Salary reviews
- Staff evaluations – by whom and when
- Salary increases
- Office rules and discipline (including policies on warning letters and termination)
- Severance pay
- Office parking policies
- Overtime
- Policy for staff conflicts
- Sick leave and sick days
- Personal days
- Tardiness
- Outside employment

- Lunch and dinner breaks
- Housekeeping
- Smoking policy
- Continuing education
- Personal phone calls
- Team meeting
- Staff dental days

Other policies you may wish to include are:

- Financial policies
- Insurance policies
- Patient policies

The entire team should be involved in drafting the office policy manual – keeping in mind that the dentist has the final say in setting all policies. The dentist should set the office policies (without the involvement of the team) for:

- Staffing, evaluations and reviews
- Termination, tardiness and absenteeism
- Staff benefits
- Staff holidays, personal days, staff dental days, etc.

One person should be in charge of typing up a rough draft for team review. Each person should participate and make comments and suggestions. The final decision on policies belongs to the dentist. When the final draft has been completed, each team member should receive their own copy to read and keep. One manual should be kept in the office at all times. Each year the office policy manual should be updated. All new employees should receive their own manual.

SAMPLE OFFICE POLICY MANUAL

The following office policy manual is a sample written exclusively for this workbook. Any similarities to persons, policies, places, etc. is purely coincidental.

Each section's information is to be used as a guideline only. Every practice is unique and individual. Therefore, your policies should reflect your own practice, systems and philosophy on patient care and employee relations. We strongly urge you to check with your provincial/state government for rules and regulations concerning termination, statutory holidays, vacation periods, notice of termination, severance pay, medical leave, working hours and overtime pay.

A Manual might be similar to the following *Sample*:

Our Office Philosophy

Our dental practice is a team-spirited, patient-centered office. We believe in the best possible care for all of our patients and will do our best to give them that care. We treat each patient exactly the same, in a friendly, caring manner, and we never pre-judge their ability to pay for services. We offer many choices and alternatives for complete comprehensive care. We continually update our skills and our technology for the benefit of our patients' care and also for our own personal and professional growth. We try our best to follow all of the outlined policies and back each other 100% with those policies.

Office and Working Hours

Our office (patient) hours are as follows:

Monday	9:00 - 3:30	6.5	hours
Tuesday	10:00 - 7:00	9.0	hours
Wednesday	8:30 - 2:30	6.0	hours
Thursday	9:00 - 5:30	8.5	hours
Friday	9:00 - 12:00	3.0	hours
Total Patient hours:		33.0	hours

Our working hours are as follows:

Monday	8:45 - 3:45	7.0	hours
Tuesday	9:45 - 7:15	9.5	hours
Wednesday	8:15 - 4:30	7.25	hours
Thursday	8:45 - 5:45	9.0	hours
Friday	8:45 - 2:00	5.25	hours
Staff Meeting	2:00 - 4:00	2.0	hours
Total Working hours:		40.0	hours

Salary Policies

Staff will be paid a weekly salary based on our working hours – not patient hours. Because all staff members will be paid with a set salary, there is no overtime pay (unless they work more than 44 hours per week and they are not in a managerial position).

Part-time staff is paid on a daily basis rather than on an hourly basis, and the above notes also apply to part-time staff. You are considered a part-time employee if you work 28 hours or less at this practice.

As a rule, we *all* leave at the same time in the evening (with the exception of

Dr. Smith, who may wish to stay later in the evening for treatment planning or administration). If you have finished your work early, please ask the other team members if they need any help and when everything is done, we will leave together. It is unfair if one or two people get to leave early all of the time.

Lunch/Dinner Breaks

Each staff member will receive no less than 30 minutes and no more than 60 minutes for lunch depending upon the day's schedule.

Personal Appearance

Dental Assistants: White, blue or pink dental uniform & white shoes.
Dental Hygienists: White, blue or pink dental uniform & white shoes.
Business Staff: Business attire such as suits, blouses or dress pants.

Make up, jewelry and perfume are fine as long as it is not overdone. We do request that if clinical staff wear nail polish, the color be clear while at work. (In some jurisdictions, it is illegal to specify clothing requirements unless a uniform or clothing allowance is provided. Check with your local branch of employment standards.)

Outside Employment

In all fairness to our patients and other staff members, your position here should be your first priority. Outside employment is fine as long as it does not interfere with our working hours or your job performance in the office.

Housekeeping

We have a cleaning company who come in nightly to clean the office. However, each person is responsible for their own area and are not to rely on the cleaning service.

Assistants and hygienists must clean their rooms between patients, which means adhering to complete infection control procedures.

The business staff are responsible for keeping all paper and files neat and orderly at all times. In addition, the desk should be wiped clean at night and all files put away before you leave in the evening.

Staff Meetings

We have regular monthly meetings and *all* staff members are expected to attend and to participate. If you are not scheduled to work on our meeting day, you are still required to attend our team meeting (for which you will be compensated). Our meetings are not complaint sessions. We discuss practice progress and concerns, new ideas, implementing new systems, etc. People-problems should be discussed privately, between the individuals directly involved – one on one.

An agenda will be posted in our staff room, listing the topics to be discussed at each session. Please feel free to add anything you would like to discuss. We will also review the production and other aspects of the previous month and how we can improve on them the next month. Any new ideas and suggestions are always welcome.

Personal Phone Calls

Personal phone calls are not permitted during working hours – except in emergency situations. If you need to make a phone call during the day, please do so on your break or at lunch time. Use only the private line for personal calls – no exceptions to this rule.

Messages will be taken for all staff members (dentists included) and you may return the calls as specified above. We ask that you keep personal calls to a minimum as this is a working environment. All calls for Dr. Smith should have a message taken, unless he specifies otherwise in the morning or he is on a break.

Answering the Telephone

Try to answer the telephone within three rings. If you are on the other line, excuse yourself for a moment and answer the ringing line. An endlessly ringing line may mean a lost patient. For all outgoing calls (insurance, collections, ordering, etc.), use the private line so that our advertised lines are free at all times.

Smoking

We are in the health profession and as such, our office is a completely smoke-free environment.

Holidays and Vacation Time

1. Staff are allowed the following number of weeks for vacation according to the number of years employed:

2 weeks	After 1 year of employment
3 weeks	Between 2 and 7 years of employment
4 weeks	Between 7 and 10 years of employment
5 weeks	Over 10 years of employment

2. Staff *must* take one week of their vacation time during the week that Dr. Smith is on vacation.
3. Staff will receive full pay for two weeks of holidays per year (this constitutes the 4% vacation pay) after one year with increases as above.
4. Vacation times are on a first-come-first-served basis. Please put into writing your specific requested week(s) of vacation and give to our office coordinator for scheduling purposes. Conflicts will be resolved based on seniority.

Office Parking

Office parking is free for our building. We request that you park your car towards the rear of the parking lot and leave the front parking spaces for our patients.

Personal and Family Dental Care

Personal Dental Care

Staff is entitled to free dentistry (although you must pay for your own lab costs). Twice each year we will set aside one full Saturday or Sunday for a staff dental day. All preventive and restorative work will be completed with the help of our team and everyone is required to attend. You will *not* be compensated for this day as all of your dental work is being performed free of charge.

Family Dental Care

Children and spouses will receive their preventive care cleanings and x-rays free. All restorative and other dental work will be billed at a 50% reduction of our regular dental fees. Lab costs are to be paid by the employee if applicable.

Personal or Mental Health Days

Staff is entitled to one personal day (floater) per year for family commitments, school plays, teacher interviews, etc. This one day must be scheduled at least *one month* in advance – in writing. This one day may be taken as two half days, but must be scheduled as specified above. You will receive your regular pay for the one day.

Sick Days and Sick Leave

Sick Days

All full-time staff members are entitled to six sick days per year with pay. Part-time staff has three paid sick days per year. You cannot build up your sick days over the year and take a vacation. The sick days are to be used only if you are ill. This office does not give bonuses, days off or pay for unused sick days.

<u>Sick Leave</u>

Staff who are off longer than three days require a doctor's note and are encouraged to file for medical leave benefits with the unemployment office. If you are ill and require a longer length of time off work, we will fill your position with a temporary employee until you are well enough to return.

Medical Appointments

We encourage you to book your medical appointments on your day off. However, if this is impossible, you will be granted time off to attend your appointment. Please give our office coordinator as much notice as possible so that we can make the necessary arrangements in the schedule.

Probationary Period

All staff members will be subject to a three-month probationary period in our office and are considered temporary employees until/if hired at the end of our three-month probationary period. During the three months, you will receive as much training as we can provide. At the end of the three months, we will schedule a doctor-employee meeting to discuss your progress and salary review – if applicable.

If, at the end of your probation period, our office does not offer you permanent employment, no notice of termination is required by law.

Salary Reviews and Staff Evaluations

<u>Staff Evaluations</u>

Each year all team members will meet privately with Dr. Smith for a staff evaluation to discuss strengths and weaknesses and how you can make any necessary improvements. Dr. Smith will also review your job expectations.

<u>Salary Reviews</u>

1. Salary reviews will be scheduled three months after your staff evaluation. Annual raises will be based on the following:
   - The results of your staff evaluation
   - Your attitude, enthusiasm and responsibilities
   - The increase in office production since your last increase
2. Raises (if applicable) will be given **once** annually. A salary review does not necessarily mean that a raise will be provided.
3. If office production has decreased (and we hope it won't!) since your last raise, raises will be suspended until the office production has increased.

Other Benefits

The following are our office benefits:

1. Two staff dental days per year.
2. 50% reduction in dental fees for family members plus complimentary preventive care appointments.
3. Two weeks paid vacation (after one year).
4. Uniform allowance of $200 per year.
5. After one year of employment, the office will pay your annual dues for membership in your local dental association. You are expected to attend the meetings if the office pays for your membership.
6. We will attend certain continuing education seminars each year and the office will pay your registration fee and hotel and meal expenses if applicable.
7. One "personal" day per year.

Continuing Education Programs

1. We will attend continuing education seminars together as a team, usually twice per year. We will decide together which programs will be appropriate and everyone is expected to attend and to take notes and bring back ideas to share with the practice.
2. If other clinical, scientific courses arise during the year, Dr. Smith will make a decision on who will attend these programs.
3. You are expected to attend your monthly association meetings if the office is paying your membership dues. The local associations often have interesting speakers and topics for discussions and it is our hope that you will learn new techniques and systems to share with our office.

Team Conflicts

If a conflict arises (and we hope it doesn't) between yourself and another team member, it is your responsibility to resolve it quietly and privately (never in front of our patients or other team members). If you are unable to resolve your conflict, Dr. Smith will arbitrate if necessary and a warning letter will be provided to each party. If the problem is not resolved, it is detrimental to our practice and Dr. Smith will take appropriate action.

Office Discipline and Termination

All staff members will receive written warnings if they do not perform their job responsibilities to our specifications and expectations. Keep in mind that Dr.

Smith will talk with you privately as well. If, after three written warnings, your job performance/attitude does not improve, your employment will be terminated and the following notice will be provided:

1 year or less:	1 week notice
2 years or less:	2 weeks notice
3 years or less:	3 weeks notice

and so on, according to the number of years worked to a maximum of 8 weeks notice. Severance pay is not applicable per se, although if your employment is terminated without notice you will be given the corresponding number of weeks of severance pay in lieu of notice.

No notice of termination will be given for the following:

1. Temporary employees of less than one year.
2. Employees who are being laid off temporarily (13 weeks or less in any 20-week period).
3. An employee who is guilty of wilful misconduct, disobedience or wilful neglect of duty that has not been condoned.
4. An employee who has refused reasonable alternative work at our office.
5. An employee who does not return from a temporary layoff within a reasonable amount of time.

Statutory Holidays

Staff members who have been employed for more than three months are entitled to pay (8 hours per day) for recognized public holidays. As statutory holidays differ according to jurisdiction, please check with your local government employment office.

Staff members will not receive pay for public holidays if:

1. They have been employed for less than three months.
2. They do not earn wages on twelve days of the four weeks preceding the holiday.
3. The employee does not work his/her regular day of work preceding or following the holiday.

Absenteeism and Tardiness

Absenteeism

As specified above, each employee is entitled to six paid sick days per year. Please call our office the evening before, if able, and leave a message on our machine if you will not be in the next day.

Tardiness

Tardiness affects many people in the office. For this reason, we ask that you make every effort to be at work at the specified time. If you will be unavoidably late, please call our office and let us know so that we can make appropriate arrangements to cover for you until you arrive. Continued tardiness will result in written warnings from Dr. Smith.

Our Patient Policies

Emergency Patient Procedures

As you are aware, emergency patients must be seen as soon as possible. First thing in the morning, we will set aside emergency patient time in the appointment book. The patient needs to be informed that this appointment will be to make a diagnosis only and relieve any discomfort. The patient will be given the next available appointment in order to complete their treatment.

Pediatric Patients

It is our policy that pediatric patients be accompanied by their parent/guardian until they are ten years old. This should be explained to parents over the telephone. Remember that the child is the patient, not the parent. Greet the child by name when they come and let them know that we were expecting them. This makes them feel more at ease. To make our job easier and to make it easier on the child, we prefer no parents or visitors in the treatment room unless Dr. Smith feels it is necessary for the comfort of the child.

We begin to see children at age three. Their first appointment consists of an office tour, a ride in the treatment chair and oral hygiene instruction. We want to provide an introduction for the children before they have their first regular prophy. For older children, we have headphones if they want to hear music during their treatment. We have a selection of cassettes or they may bring their own.

Geriatric/Special Needs Patients

Some of these patients may require our assistance up and down stairs, or into the chair, and perhaps to complete our forms. Treat our elderly patients with respect and remember that everyone deserves our time and consideration.

Late Patients

If a patient is only slightly late, we will perform what treatment we can with the time remaining in their appointments, then reschedule another appointment to complete treatment, so as not to keep our other patients waiting. If the patient is very late, they will need to reschedule their appointment in all fairness to others.

No-Show Patients

If a patient does not show, call them immediately to reschedule. If you cannot reach them, make a note on your pending appointment list for calling. If a patient does not show twice, they will receive a letter stating that in the future, they will have to call our office the day prior to their scheduled appointment to confirm that they will be there. If they do not call, we will schedule another patient in their place.

Difficult Patients

Difficult patients should be dealt with in a calm, friendly manner. Many times an angry patient who is confronted by calmness will in turn calm down. However, if the patient becomes verbally abusive or begins to shout in front of others, please show him/her to my office and I will deal with the problem personally.

Our Financial Policies

1. Treatment less than $100.00 is due at the time of treatment by cash, check, post-dated check, direct deposit or credit card (e.g., Visa and MasterCard).
2. As a rule, we do not accept assignment of insurance. However, if a patient is experiencing financial difficulty, we will do so. They must pay the out-of-pocket portion of insurance at the time of treatment or make financial arrangements to pay it.
3. We make written financial arrangements for patients. Our Financial Coordinator will handle this in our consultation room.
4. The out-of-pocket portion of insurance is always due at the time of treatment. If this amount is large, we would be happy to make financial arrangements with the patient.
5. When we receive a predetermination back from the insurance company, it is our policy to call the patient immediately to let them know of their insurance coverage.
6. It is office policy to telephone overdue accounts rather than send a statement. Most people ignore statements but they cannot ignore the person on the telephone.
7. We always discuss fees with patients before treatment begins. Our Financial Coordinator will discuss fees in the consultation room if it is for extensive

treatment. For fillings and basic restoratives, the receptionist will let the patient know the fee when they schedule an appointment to complete restorative work. If the patient requires financial arrangements, please refer them to our Financial Coordinator.

8. The patient should always be advised that dental insurance is a contract between his/her employer and the insurance company. If any disputes arise concerning dental insurance, the patient should advise their employer or contact their insurance company directly. Insurance disputes are not the concern of our office unless we have filled the form out incorrectly (which we never do!?!).

SUMMARY

- These policies are samples only.
- Dental office policies must be concise and clear so that each employee has a clear understanding of the rules in your dental practice.
- It is much better to have your policies in writing to avoid disappointments and frustrations.
- All employees should have a copy of the office policy manual.
- All manuals should be updated on a yearly basis to keep up with the times.
- The most important thing to remember when compiling your manual is that you must check with the employment standards agency in your area for regulations on termination, holidays, working hours, etc. Please ensure that your office policy manual is within the guidelines of your state/ provincial laws.
- Keep your policies basic, simple to understand and easy to implement.

AREAS OUR PRACTICE CAN IMPROVE UPON

NOTES

FIGURE 4.1 SAMPLE: TEAM MEETING AGENDA AND GUIDELINES

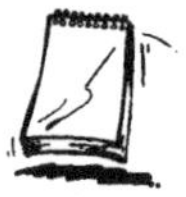

Month:_____

Date of Meeting:_____

Staff Members in Attendance:_____

_____

	PREVIOUS MONTH	THIS MONTH	DIFFERENCE
Doctor(s) Production			
Hygiene Production			
Other Production			
Total Production			
Collections			
New Patients			
No Shows			
T.U. of Down Time			
Cancellations			

Old Business:

1._____

2._____

3._____

4._____

New Business:

1._____

2._____

3._____

4._____

Clinical Team Report:_____

Business Team Report:_____

_____

4.
TEAM MEETINGS

"There is no I in team."
Unknown

TEAM MEETING GUIDELINES

1. Team meetings should be held on a regular basis, at least one per month for two hours of uninterrupted time. Individuals can also hold departmental meetings on a more regular basis (e.g., hygiene department, business department) if you have a large practice.

2. If meetings take place after work, staff should be paid for their time. Or, if part-time staff attends on an unscheduled day, they should be compensated for their time. When you pay people for their time, you should expect and get participation.

3. Each and every person on the staff should make every effort to attend the monthly staff meeting, including the dentist and all associates. Practice success is a team effort.

4. Appoint one person as a facilitator for the meeting (to lead the discussion). The facilitator should be changed for each meeting so that everyone on the team has a chance to lead a meeting. Make sure that everyone on your team is comfortable leading a meeting; if not, don't force them.

5. Always document your team meetings for later referral. You can document the meeting with an audio tape, a video tape or by writing down comments. If a staff member was sick or unable to attend, you have a reference for them. You can use figure 4.1 as a sample Team Meeting Agenda and Guideline.

6. The facilitator should start the meeting by commenting on all the things the team is doing well. Everyone should be encouraged to comment.

7. Each person should give a report on their area of practice. For example, the appointment secretary can comment on down time, cancellations, new patient numbers, etc.

FIGURE 4.2 SAMPLE: TEAM MEETING PROGRESS PLANNER

MONTH: _____

New Business/Ideas	Person(s) in Charge	Method/How to Plan	Deadline Date	☑
1				
2				
3				
4				
5				
6				

8.   Review the previous month's meeting notes: Did we reach our goals? Did we make the changes discussed? If not, why? Do we need more time? Did we encourage each other? Never point fingers or lay blame – you just need to have the facts so that you can move ahead.

9.   Check off the tasks which were completed and start the meeting with topics which had to be carried over. Add on new business, topics and suggestions. As a new topic is discussed, everyone should listen and then weigh the pros and cons of the new idea. Four heads are better than one for generating ideas.

10. Once you have made a decision related to new ideas, you must assign responsibility to team members who will be accountable for following through with the new idea. List:
   • Who will make this happen? Support person?
   • How will they do it?
   • What is the deadline date for completion? Time required?
   • Obstacles, if any?
   Use a Team Meeting Progress Planner (see figure 4.2). The Progress Planner can help you document new ideas and bring tasks to a conclusion.

11. When all topics have been covered, you should focus on setting new goals for the following month. Goals may include: plans for reducing down time, production goals, collection goals, new patient numbers, increasing staff motivation, continuing education courses to attend.

12. Take advantage of creative and/or artistic team members. These people are usually great at helping with new marketing ideas and newsletters.

Team meetings should be productive and organized, a time to share ideas and network with your co-workers. I have met many dentists and staff who just want to be heard. They want encouragement; they want to share their new ideas and grow personally and professionally.

If you can make your staff meetings productive and tension-free, everyone will benefit. Your patients will have a more positive environment, as will the entire team. It is okay to have fun, to plan something unique. Have fun at your meetings and give praise where praise is due.

ANNUAL FULL-DAY MEETINGS

Once per year each dental office should take a full day to hold a team meeting and to reorganize for the coming year. Usually the best time is the end of August or beginning of September as this marks the beginning of the new school year and the end of vacations and holidays. Everyone is just getting back into a normal work mode.

Your yearly meeting is essential for reorganizing business areas and setting new goals. Topics to be discussed at an annual full-day meeting include:

- Patient Service: Which areas can you improve upon to make your patient's visit more comfortable and enjoyable?

- Continuing Education: Which programs would you like to attend? Which out of town convention? Who gets to go? How can you budget for continuing education?

- Staffing Requirements: Do you currently have enough staff to handle the day-to-day tasks in your practice? Will a new team member fit into your budget? Are you going to expand your hygiene program?

- New Production Goals: Although each practice should be setting monthly production goals, a yearly total allows you to see the big picture.

- Office Design: Does your office need a new coat of paint? New wallpaper, plants, pictures?

- Business Systems: Are your systems fully productive and organized? How efficient is your collection system? Recall system? Insurance and predeterminations? What changes will be necessary in the coming year?

- New Equipment: All practices have to update at some point. Take a look at your current equipment and decide what you need to replace and where the funds will come from – budget, financing, etc.

- Computers: If you are not already computerized, discuss the benefits of a computer system. If your practice is computerized, you may wish to discuss upgrading your system, deciding if you need additional terminals or updated software.

- Marketing Plans: The yearly meeting is a great time to set out a marketing plan for the coming year. Decide what your budget is and what type of marketing ideas you want to implement.

- Review of Last Year's Figures: This includes new patient numbers, cancelled appointments, no-shows and production/collection figures. Discuss the areas in which you need to improve. How can you improve those figures?

Make your annual full-day meeting fun. Order lunch for the entire team or hold your meeting in a hotel meeting room for a change. The idea is to keep your meeting positive, enthusiastic and motivating. This is a new year for all of you – a time to make plans to move toward the future.

DO'S AND DON'TS FOR TEAM MEETINGS

DO NOT:

- Put a message on your bulletin board, *"All firings will continue until morale improves"*.
- Pick on the dentist(s) or other staff members. Never place blame on others – especially in front of the entire team. Instead, offer constructive comments and try to help others overcome their weaknesses by offering solutions instead of complaints.
- Complain about money. If you want a raise or cannot pay the payables on time, take it up with the dentist in private.
- Make statements such as, *"Things are so bad you might not even have a job next month"* . Try to keep morale high.
- Criticize others. Team meetings should not be gripe sessions, they should be productive discussions about the practice.
- Sulk or look bored (even if you are!). Looking bored demotivates others and shows the rest of the staff that you are not a team player. Even if the current discussion does not involve you or your position, you can still join in the discussion and offer your own ideas or at least listen attentively.
- Dominate the conversation. Listening is one of the best ways to communicate. Give everyone on the team a chance to voice their own opinions and ideas.
- Think only your suggestions are worth talking about. Everyone gives their own unique contribution to the practice. Discuss all ideas openly.
- Dictate. Give everyone a chance to discuss ideas.
- Use negative body language (sigh, cross arms, roll eyes). This is a great way to demotivate the meeting and lower the morale of the team.

DO:

- Motivate people by being positive.
- Encourage all team members to attend. Each person makes up a part of the team and all staff play an important role in the running of the practice.
- Make sure that staff who were unable to attend receive a copy of the meeting notes.
- Always thank people for suggestions.
- Give praise and appreciation for a job well done. Appreciation boosts self-confidence.
- Give a report on your area of the practice to keep everyone informed.

- Review the previous month's statistics.
- Set new goals.
- Discuss new projects.
- Listen attentively to all suggestions.
- Post a list of topics to be discussed – which everyone can add to.
- Document your meetings (audio tape, video or written) for referral.
- Take turns facilitating the meetings.
- Remember each team member is valuable – recognize their individual contribution to the practice.

MORNING MEETINGS

Each practice should hold morning meetings on a daily basis. Everyone should be encouraged to attend (dentists included) and to be on time. The morning meeting will set the tone for the day, so make yours positive.

TOPICS FOR DISCUSSION AT A MORNING MEETING:
- Which patients will be in for treatment today? Which of those patients requires special care?
- Are there any openings that need to be filled?
- Are all premedicated patients taking their medication?
- Are all lab cases back from the lab in time for the patients' appointments?
- Where will emergency patients fit into the schedule?
- Do any staff members need help with duties?
- Identify the new patients for the day.

DOCTOR-TO-DOCTOR MEETINGS

If you have an associate(s) or a partner(s), regular meetings between principals should be scheduled on a monthly basis. In order to stay on top of administration duties and organization of the practice, some systems must be monitored. If your office has a practice administrator or coordinator, this person should also attend.

Items on the meeting agenda should include:
- Financial aspects of the practice which need to be addressed, such as

banking, monthly reconciliations, production, loans, interest, mutual investments, accounts payables, etc.
- Staffing requirements/problems.
- Practice planning such as marketing budgets, office expansion, new equipment or procedures.
- Upcoming continuing education programs or conferences.
- Working schedules for the next month.

SUMMARY

- Regular, productive staff meetings are a must on a monthly basis.
- Every staff member must make every effort to attend staff meetings.
- All staff members should be financially compensated for meetings during which they are not scheduled to work.
- Always have a meeting agenda which staff can add to during the month.
- Document your meeting for easy referral.
- Assign tasks and completion dates.
- Participate openly and professionally. Don't place blame or pick on other team members.

AREAS OUR PRACTICE CAN IMPROVE UPON

NOTES

"Before everything else, getting ready is the secret of success."
Henry Ford

5.

INCENTIVES FOR THE DENTAL TEAM

Success has a direct relationship between employee job satisfaction and how much the employee feels a part of the dental practice. As a business owner, you need to ask yourself, *"What is the benefit to my employee to work here?"* Money alone is not always the biggest motivator, although it is close as people need money to meet their needs and maintain a comfortable lifestyle. Big motivators for employees include (in no particular order):

- Recognition at work: the feeling that the employer recognizes their unique contribution to the dental practice.
- A good salary to maintain a comfortable lifestyle.
- Personal and professional growth on the job.
- Praise and appreciation from the dentist that they are doing a good job.
- Responsibility. Most people want to feel that they are responsible and accountable for doing a good job.

If your employees are responsible for increased practice profit, they often need to know, *"How will I benefit from this increased profit?"* An incentive bonus, given over and above the employees' salary, provides your team member with an extra source of motivation to be even more productive and industrious.

My preference is not a monthly bonus based on production goals (although the production goals are very important). Sometimes a regular monthly bonus becomes expected and taken for granted. I prefer a nice, surprise bonus given when least expected. I have included the guidelines for incentives based on production for those dentists who prefer them. Other forms of incentives follow in this chapter.

- A note to dentists – Incentive bonuses or any type of bonuses are not mandatory. If you are not comfortable giving bonuses, then please don't. This chapter is provided for dentists interested in providing incentives.

INCENTIVE BONUS PLANS BASED ON PRODUCTION

By far, the most popular form of incentive is a monetary reward based on increased production numbers. However, many practices set a production goal that is unattainable or give such a big bonus that the dentist feels miserable about giving the check. Production goals must be realistic or else you will demotivate yourself and your team. Financial rewards must be within the practice's budget or the dentist will come to resent giving the bonus. Both situations are bad for the team member and the dentist. In order to create a comfortable, reasonable bonus based on production, please refer to the following guidelines:

1. Your collection percentage must be above 96%. There is no point in giving team members a bonus based on production if you are not going to collect all of the revenue you have produced and worked so hard for. Collection ratios should remain above this level for at least three months before you go ahead with any type of incentive bonus plan.

2. Your monthly production goal must be realistic. If your average monthly production is $25,000, it would be unrealistic and unfair to employees to set a goal of $40,000 per month. A more realistic goal would be to increase your monthly production by an amount that is attainable and realistic.

3. Before increasing your production goal, the previous goal should be met for at least 2 to 4 months in order to ensure that you can in fact remain at this level of production. (The employee still receives a bonus each of these months if the goal is met). The dentist should decide when it is time to increase the production goal. I wouldn't recommend any longer than 4 months.

4. The monetary rewards should be exactly the same for each full-time employee. Part-time employees should be pro-rated according to the number of hours per week they work. Any type of favoritism promotes low morale and competition. Each team member is a contributor to the practice regardless of whether or not they are a producer. The dental receptionist must produce a well scheduled appointment book so that the clinical team can be productive. She must also ensure that your collection

percentage remains above 96%. Your hygienist is a producer who creates revenue. Dental assistants help the dentist to work faster by assisting with patients, room clean-up, sterilization and more. Everyone contributes to the success of a dental practice and therefore the rewards for all should be the same.

5. The only exception to this rule is when you hire a new employee. If your practice has been reaching your production goals for the past 6 months and the monthly bonus has increased by $30, the new employee should receive the bonus that everyone else started with. The new employee bonus should increase by the same monthly amount as the rest of the team.

6. If your monthly goal is not reached, there should be no bonus. If you start to give out bonuses regardless of whether a goal has been reached, it will be taken for granted and expected. This is not motivating, nor is it productive. An incentive bonus based on goals is provided only when the goal is reached.

SETTING A MONETARY AMOUNT

Far too many doctors give a large bonus. If you set the dollar amount too high and increase it by large amounts each time you reach a goal, you will be setting yourself up for big headaches. I recommend the following monetary rewards:

*   **Full-time employees:** $50.00/month with an increase of $10.00/month each time the goal is raised and met.
*   **Part-time employees:** $25.00/month with an increase of $5.00/month each time the goal is raised and met.

This does not seem like a great deal of money at first but it can build up quickly. For example, let's look at this over the time span of one year with 5 full-time employees who meet their goal each month.

January	Goal met	$50 x 5 employees = $250.00
February	Goal met	$50 x 5 employees = $250.00
March	Increased goal met	$60 x 5 employees = $300.00
April	Goal met	$60 x 5 employees = $300.00
May	Goal met	$60 x 5 employees = $300.00
June	Increased goal met	$70 x 5 employees = $350.00

July	Goal met	$70 x 5 employees = $350.00
August	Increased goal met	$80 x 5 employees = $400.00
September	Goal met	$80 x 5 employees = $400.00
October	Goal met	$80 x 5 employees = $400.00
November	Increased goal met	$90 x 5 employees = $450.00
December	Goal met	$90 x 5 employees = $450.00

Total Bonus for Year = $4,200.00

For that one year the total bonus paid is $4,200. This is fine because your production has increased and the practice is making more money. However, once you get 3 or 4 years into the bonus plan, each employee (if you have a low staff turnover) will be receiving a bonus of approximately $200/month. If you still have 5 employees, your monthly expenditures for bonuses will be $1000/month or $12,000 per year (this is based on the assumption that you are meeting each monthly goal).

Each doctor should weigh carefully the pros and cons of an incentive bonus plan based on production increases (this is where good procrastination skills come in). Another aspect to carefully consider is how long will you stay with this type of incentive bonus. Remember that something received on a regular basis is not given up easily.

If you decide to go with the monthly bonus, set a maximum amount. Once that amount is reached, the bonus remains the same. Your team members should be informed of the maximum amount before you begin the incentive plan. It is up to each practice to decide upon the maximum amount; however, I would recommend that the bonus go no higher than $150 per month. I have seen far too many dentists struggling to hand out a bonus check of $300 - $400 to five employees every month.

Some dentists prefer to pay a bonus at the year end based on a percentage of the profit. Often staff lose interest waiting a year for a bonus. Staff should be informed that bonuses are taxable, sometimes at a higher rate. Check with your local jurisdiction for current information.

CONTINUING EDUCATION AS AN INCENTIVE BONUS

Continuing education programs not only benefit the team member, they also benefit the practice. Most people love to go on continuing education courses as it gives them a break from the office and a chance to grow personally as well as professionally. It is also a great opportunity for networking with one's peers.

TIPS FOR EDUCATION AS AN INCENTIVE

1. Let each team member decide, on a yearly basis, the programs they would like to attend (of course the dentist makes the final decision) if the practice goals are reached.
2. The practice goals do not necessarily have to focus on production. Other goals may include:
   - Increasing the new patient numbers on a monthly basis.
   - Reducing the number of no-shows on a monthly basis.
   - Increasing case acceptance of elective dentistry.

   Decide what your goal will be and set it in writing so that each team member fully understands the goals and the rewards.
3. If the goal is reached, the team member can attend the continuing education program.
4. To make continuing education more of an incentive, the program should have added bonuses for the employee such as lunch included. A major convention is always a great motivator for dental team members. They can walk around the exhibits, sit in on a number of programs, have lunch as a team. If the conference is in another city, it is like a trip for most employees. Going together as a team is a great motivator for increasing team spirit.

I think continuing education is a great incentive bonus for any type of practice. Everyone benefits.

OTHER FORMS OF INCENTIVE BONUSES

Personally, I prefer a combination of the continuing education incentive with surprise bonuses throughout the year. Surprises can take many forms (listed below) and are usually not expected. The surprise bonuses cannot be taken for granted because one never knows when they are coming.
- An occasional cash bonus is impromptu and unexpected, *"My way of saying thank you for doing such a great job"*. The amount need not be high.

- Tickets to a play or a sports event.
- Take your entire staff for a nice lunch as a surprise.
- Buy your staff membership to a local gym or fitness club.
- Paid time off in the summer. On all long weekends, give your team the extra Friday or Monday off so that they have a four-day weekend instead of three. They should be paid for this day as it is a bonus.
- Shorter working hours in the summer with the same pay. Instead of leaving at 5:00 pm on a Friday, leave at 3:30 or 4:00 pm and pay your staff for this time anyway.
- Bonuses given at Christmas are sometimes expected. I believe Christmas is for giving, but giving from the heart, not from the pocket book. A nice dinner at a fancy restaurant with a suitable gift for each employee is an excellent treat. A monetary bonus is usually appreciated as long as you are comfortable with it.
- Flexibility with working hours is a great incentive. Many team members have small children. Grant them the extra time off (with pay) to go and see their child's Christmas concert or play or a teacher's interview. The half day or so that they will be gone, you can cover with other team members – this is what team work is all about.

Never give a bonus to employees who are not doing a good job or who are miserable all the time. These people should not even be in your practice. The main reason for a bonus or an incentive is to reward and motivate excellent, team spirited staff members. I give incentives happily to my team, but I do expect to be rewarded with hard work, commitment and loyalty.

AREAS OUR PRACTICE CAN IMPROVE UPON

NOTES

6.

THE HYGIENE DEPARTMENT AND PERIODONTAL PROGRAMS

The hygiene department is the life of the general practice. An organized and productive recall center will be the catalyst for increased case acceptance of comprehensive care. Therefore, organization and set systems for the hygiene department are necessary.

Before we discuss periodontal programs, let's review the different types of preventive care programs in dentistry.

1. **TELEPHONE RECALL PROGRAM**

   A hygiene maintenance program via the telephone will work well for many practices if organized and detailed with a back-up system for patients. The patients are called by the dental office to schedule an appointment when they are due for their next hygiene appointment.

2. **POSTCARD RECALL PROGRAM**

   The postcard system is an old-fashioned and increasingly obsolete way of organizing the dental recall program – especially in this age of computerization. Although many practices still use this system, it is the least effective and has the most disadvantages. When a patient is due for a hygiene appointment, the dental office sends out a recall postcard with the general message, *"It's time for your appointment. Call our office to schedule"*. The onus is on the patient to respond rather than the practice. Generally, only about one-quarter of patients respond.

3. **PREAPPOINTING RECALL PROGRAM**

   Preappointing recall patients is an excellent system which works best with detailed follow-up and continuity. The preappointing can be done either by the front desk team or by the hygienist(s). A chairside computer with the schedule may also be used by the hygienist.

Ideally, the preappointing method works best. Not all patients will preappoint (though most will if your team uses the proper communication skills), so a combination of preappointing and the telephone system is the most effective method for recall systems. The advantages include:

- Patients are committed to the practice if the hygienist takes the time to explain to patients why they need to return on a regular basis.
- Saves a considerable amount of time for the business team. Fewer telephone calls are made trying to get people in for recall appointments as about 75% of your patients will preappoint.
- Cuts down on costs related to staff salaries (many practices hire extra staff for recall calls only).
- Personal contact with patients right in the office.
- Can reinforce the importance of professional care for the next appointment while the patient is making their next appointment.
- Saves on the paperwork for the business team.

Before implementing any type of periodontal program, your recall system must be as effective as possible. Consider the following:

> You have 1,400 active patients, each of whom should be seen twice each year. You have the potential for 2,800 recall appointments per year or approximately 230 patients per month. If your hygienist sees 10 patients per day, five days per week for one month (22 working days), she will have seen 220 patients. This recall system would be 96% effective.

The formula for recall system effectiveness is:

Part I
1. Take the number of active patients you have and double that number (2 recall appointments per year).
2. Divide this number by 12 (12 months).

Part II
1. Calculate how many patients your hygienist(s) sees on an average day.
2. Calculate how many days your hygienist(s) works each month.
3. Multiply the number of patients seen per day by the number of hygiene days per month.

Part III
1. Divide the answer obtained in part II by the answer from part I and this will give you a percentage of effectiveness in your recall program.

SAMPLE:
- 1,850 active patients x 2 = 3700
- 3,700 ÷ 12 = **308**
- 9 patients seen per day (average)
- 22 days per month
- 12 x 22 = **198**
- 198 ÷ 308 = 0.642 or **64%** effective

These figures should be monitored for at least three months to determine the average effectiveness of your recall program over a period of time. It is recommended that before you implement a periodontal program in your practice, your recall system should be effective.

PERIODONTAL PROGRAMS FOR GENERAL PRACTICE

Statistics inform us that 8 out of 10 adults have some form of periodontal disease during their lifetime. Yet, a low percentage of hygiene appointments are for periodontal conditions. Why not offer your patients the option of complete hygiene care? Allow them to decide if they want to make the investment to keep their teeth for a lifetime.

Your patients need to know if they are a regular preventive care patient or if they have some form (class I - IV) of periodontal disease. Don't be too shy to mention disease, gum infection, swelling, bleeding – all of those terms help our patients understand that tooth loss and/or bone loss may result from neglect.

The goals of the periodontal program include:
- Retention of the patient's natural dentition in use and in comfort.
- Stopping the advance of periodontal disease.
- Preventing recurrence of periodontal disease.
- Providing your patient with quality care and service.

Setting up a periodontal program in general practice must be done with thorough research, organization and team work. Before deciding to go ahead and perform perio work on patients, you must have a set system in place. To organize your system, consider the following:

1. *When will you begin the program?*
   Set a deadline date to complete your research, organization and have the system set up and ready to go.

2. *Who will be in charge of implementing your system?*
   Ideally, your hygienist(s) should be in charge of the perio program – with the dentist's input and final say of course. The hygienists are the ones who will be completing much of the general treatment for patients.

3. *Do you have enough staff to implement the perio program?*
   You must consider that there will be extra duties involved for all team members. Hygienists will be seeing more patients, as will the dentist. The business team will have additional paperwork and scheduling responsibilities to consider.

4. *Do you have the space to implement your perio program?*
   Keep in mind that you will still be seeing recall patients regularly. Therefore, another treatment room for perio patients will become necessary as the perio program increases in size and scope over time.

5. *Do you have the extra time necessary for a perio program?*
   As the dentist, you will be examining and treating many of the perio patients yourself. If your schedule is already full, are you ready to increase your hours or to hire an associate dentist?

6. *How much money will it cost to implement your perio program?*
   The costs to consider include:
   - Perio treatment planning forms
   - Additional staff salaries once the program is up and running
   - Additional paperwork costs to cover
   - The possible added expense of another treatment room
   - Instruments and other necessary equipment and supplies

7. *Do you know a respected periodontist to refer patients to?*
   There will be patients who must be sent to a periodontist. The idea of the periodontal program is not to make a general practitioner into a specialist, but to provide a cost-effective, quality service to patients in need of general periodontal treatment at their family practice. You must have a periodontist to whom you can refer patients who clinically require perio services.

Benefits of a Perio Referral Program

Often patients are referred to a periodontist without realizing they have a problem or without being informed by their general dentist that there was a concern about periodontal disease, bone loss or possible tooth loss.

Patients often prefer to remain with their general dentist rather than to be referred – that is their choice.

The advantages of a referral program are:

- Patient awareness
- Promotes quality dentistry
- Reinforces the importance of keeping your teeth for a lifetime
- Promotes specialized dentistry

THE ORGANIZATION OF PERIODONTAL PROGRAMS

In order to maintain a productive periodontal program, organization in both the administrative and clinical areas is necessary to ensure success.

ADMINISTRATIVE AREAS

1. **Fees**

   The first step to be taken in the administrative area is to set your fees for each type of periodontal treatment you will be offering patients. The fees you set should be cost effective (to both your practice and the patient) and consistent. Fees should always remain consistent. It is far easier to quote set fees than fees which are subject to change at the doctor's discretion. It is recommended that you follow the current fee guide for your area. You are running a business and are in business to make a profit. Making a profit does not mean you are overcharging or running an assembly line. Quality patient care can be provided while still increasing production.

2. **Insurance Codes**

   It is vital that you have organized your insurance system and predetermination system to accommodate patients in the periodontal program. You must have set codes for each procedure much like the regular recall appointment. Front desk teams should have this information prior to the commencement of your perio program.

   Unfortunately, some insurance policies do not cover periodontal programs. Others cover only a portion of the treatment. It is important that your patients know that treatment may not be covered before you proceed with treatment. If the treatment is not covered, it is important to make written financial arrangements with the patient.

3. **Scheduling**

   As always, the appointment book is vital to the success of the practice. A well-scheduled day should be productive and as stress-free as possible. For the periodontal program, you should decide beforehand the appointment times for each procedure (although they may vary somewhat for individual patients). These should be listed and given to your front desk team so that they can schedule accordingly and productively.

4. **Paperwork**

   Before you begin periodontal treatment on patients, there are a number of forms and letters which you should have to increase administrative organization and legally protect your practice.

   A   Signed consent form to proceed with perio treatment. (figure 6.1)

   B   Signed form stating the patient's refusal to undergo periodontal treatment. (figure 6.2)

   C   Letter to perio patients informing them of their financial obligations. (figure 6.3)

   D   Letter confirming treatment and fees for consenting patients. (figure 6.4)

   E   Written financial arrangements and treatment. (figure 6.5)

   Samples have been provided for you to use as guidelines. It is highly recommended that you use all of the above forms and letters in your periodontal program. You must make every effort to legally protect yourself. Refer to your dental association for current rules.

5. **Marketing Your Program**

   Although the vast majority of marketing your perio program will be internal (patient education), you should also recognize the need to market externally. This does not mean placing a huge Yellow Pages advertisement. External marketing should be minor and tasteful – a notice in your newsletter and in your patient information brochure. Internal marketing includes patient education videos about periodontal disease, which should be available in your practice, as should patient education brochures. Patient education will be the most important factor for periodontal program success. We will discuss this later in the chapter.

CLINICAL AREAS

1. **Instruments and Equipment**

   Be certain that you have the necessary instruments and equipment to run a

FIGURE 6.1 SAMPLE: CONSENT FORM
TO PROCEED WITH PERIODONTAL TREATMENT

Dr. Thomas Pearson
75 Centennial Crescent Toronto Ontario M5C 2C5
(416) 555-3243
PERIODONTAL TREATMENT CONSENT FORM

Patient's Name: Mrs. Josephine Costanza
Address: 20 Mildred Court, Toronto, Ontario M6S 2V4
Telephone - Home: (416) 555-9811 **Office:**
Date: April 24, 1996

Dear Mrs. Costanza,

You have been diagnosed with Periodontal (gum) Disease. Your classification of Periodontal Disease is Class II, **which is** Mild Periodontitis. **I have outlined the following treatment necessary to combat Periodontal Disease.**

Treatment	Appointment
Scaling, Root Planing, Home Care Instruction (Quadrants 1 & 2)	45 minutes
Scaling, Root Planing, Home Care Instruction (Quadrants 3 & 4)	45 minutes
Re-examination, Prophylaxis, Probing/Charting, Evaluation	60 minutes

Please note that should you ignore your Periodontal Disease, you may have major oral health problems in the future. I have informed you of the consequences of not completing Perio treatment.

Dentistry is not a precise science. Therefore, adjustments in your periodontal treatment may have to be made which differ from the above. You will be informed of any changes before treatment commences and why those changes will be necessary.

Periodontal treatment is a combined effort of the patient and the dentist. You must realize that success depends not only on the treatment given, but on your willingness to commit to a schedule of home care. Unfortunately, there are no guarantees that treatment will succeed in improving your periodontal condition. There is a risk of failure or recurrence which you and I have discussed.

Please certifiy (signature) that you have read and understood this form and have had the periodontal treatment and associated risks explained to you. Please sign below to accept the proposed Periodontal Treatment.

Signature	Printed Name	Date

| Witness | | Thomas Pearson, D.D.S. |

FIGURE 6.2 SAMPLE: REFUSAL TO
UNDERGO PERIODONTAL TREATMENT

Dr. Heather Michaels

**987 Navigator Crescent
Regina, Saskatchewan
S1S 1S1
(306) 555-3551**

Patient Name: _____
Address: _____
Phone Number: _____
Date: _____

I,_____, have been diagnosed with periodontal
disease by Dr. Heather Michaels and do not wish to undergo Periodontal Treatment.

Dr. Michaels has explained the risks involved in neglecting periodontal treatment. The
treatment plan and alternate options of treatment have been explained to me. I understand
the risk involved with not completing prescribed treatment (possible loss of gum/teeth/bone).

I fully understand the above risks to my total health and release Dr. Heather Michaels from
any liability regarding my oral health and condition.

_____   _____   _____
Signature   **Printed Name**   **Date**

_____   _____
Witness   **Dr. Heather Michaels**

FIGURE 6.3 SAMPLE: INSURANCE PATIENTS
IN THE PERIO PROGRAM

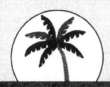

October 27, 1995

Mrs. H. Charest
23 East Exmoor Street
Orlando, FL 010101

Dear Mrs. Charest,

We are very pleased that you decided to undergo the necessary Periodontal Treatment. Any form of peridontal disease should be treated to help avoid the possible loss of teeth. Our program works in two ways. At the office, we will treat you according to the treatment plan enclosed. At home, it is your responsibility to maintain a structured home care program to ensure the best possible chance of success. Dalia, our dental hygienist, will be instructing you in home perio care at each of your appointments. By working together, we will increase the chance of success.

As we discussed at your treatment evaluation, your dental insurance will not cover the full amount of our periodontal program fees. Our office policy is to receive payment at the time of treatment directly from our patients. Your insurance coverage will be paid to you directly by the insurance company. Please fell free to call our practice any time if you have questions or would like to discuss your treatment. I look forward to seeing you soon.

Sincerely,

Dr. Mitch Hesse
enc/treatment plan

FIGURE 6.4 SAMPLE: CONFIRMATION OF
TREATMENT AND FEES

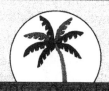

October 27, 1995

Ms. Marilyn Hampston
476 Rocklar Avenue
Orlando, FL 010101

Dear Ms. Hampston,

We are very pleased that you decided to undergo the necessary Periodontal Treatment. Any
form of peridontal disease should be treated to help avoid the possible loss of teeth. Our
program works in two ways. At the office, we will treat you according to the treatment
plan enclosed. At home, it is your responsibility to maintain a structured home care
program to ensure the best possible chance of success. Dalia, our dental hygienist, will be
instructing you in home perio care at each of your appointments. By working together, we
will increase the chance of success.

Your treatment will consist of 4 separate appointments for scaling and root planing. A re-
evaluation will then be scheduled at this time. Your total fee for this treatment is $_____.

Please feel free to call our practice any time if you have questions or would like to discuss
your treatment. I look forward to seeing you soon.

Sincerely,

Dr. Mitch Hesse

FIGURE 6.5 SAMPLE: FINANCIAL ARRANGEMENTS
AND TREATMENT

Jacob Webster, D.M.D.
105-6900 Jasper Avenue
Edmonton Alberta T5N 5N5 (403) 555-1117

Preventive & Restorative Dentistry

FINANCIAL ARRANGEMENTS FORM

PATIENT NAME: _____

ADDRESS: _____

CITY/PROV/PCODE: _____

TELEPHONE: _____

DATE: _____

Treatment	Appointment	Fee
Scaling Root Planing (Quadrant 1)	45 minutes	$---
Scaling Root Planing (Quadrant 2)	45 minutes	$---
Scaling Root Planing (Quadrant 3)	45 minutes	$---
Scaling Root Planing (Quadrant 4)	45 minutes	$---
Re-evaluation, probing/charting, prophy	60 minutes	$---
Total Fee		$---

I elect to make a deposit of $_____ on my first appointment, and pay
the balance in three monthly installments of $_____ for which I will leave
postdated checks.

_____   _____   _____
Signature   Printed Name   Date

one copy is retained by the office, the other is given to the patient

successful periodontal program. These items should be accounted for in your inventory system.

2. **Dental Chairs and Treatment Rooms**

   When you begin your program, it will be small, with few patients. However, the perio program will grow and eventually another treatment chair may be necessary. It is important to remember that you will still have regular recall patients to treat as well as patients with other procedures. Don't encourage your perio program to grow if you do not have the room to treat the patients. You could choose to refer more patients to a periodontist.

3. **Training for Clinical Team Members**

   You cannot allow your hygienist(s) to treat perio patients without the proper training. A staff training schedule should be set for the dentist to train all involved clinical team members so that there is a team philosophy and a clear understanding of the importance of the program. A continuing education course on periodontal programs would be beneficial to everyone on your team. There are many available.

GENERAL PERIODONTAL PROGRAM

Most perio programs follow similar formats and appointing schedules. Here is a sample periodontal program common to most general practices. We have not included the symptoms for each classification, as these are common knowledge to the dentist and most clinical team members. The number of appointments suggested here will vary from patient to patient depending upon individual needs.

Periodontal Classifications	Treatment Options	Appointment Time
Class I - Gingivitis	*General Practice Program*	*3 Appointments*
	•1st appointment for exam, probing and charting, x-rays and home care instructions.	• 60 minutes
	• 2nd appointment for perio scaling and home care instruction. Most patients will require only one appointment for perio scaling at this stage.	• 40 - 60 minutes

• Final appointment for probing and charting, prophy and home care instructions. If the patient has improved, they can be placed back on a regular recall program.	• 40 - 60 minutes

Class II-
Mild Periodontitis

General Practice Program	*4 - 6 Appointments*
• 1st appointment for exam, probing and charting, x-rays and home care instructions.	• 60 minutes
• 2nd - 5th appointments for perio scaling, root planing and home care instruction. Some practices prefer to scale 2 quadrants at one visit while others prefer one quadrant per visit.	• 30 - 60 minutes
• Final appointment for probing and charting, prophy and home care instructions. If the patient has improved, they can be placed back in the regular recall program and their perio condition monitored regularly. If the patient's condition has not improved, more advanced treatment or additional root planing may become necessary.	• 40 - 60 minutes

Class III-
Moderate Periodontitis

General Practice Program or Referral to a Periodontist	*6 Appointments*
• 1st appointment for exam, probing and charting, x-rays and home care instructions.	• 60 minutes
• 2nd - 5th appointments for perio scaling, root planing and home care instruction. One quadrant per visit.	• 40 - 60 minutes

• Final appointment for probing and charting, prophy, evaluation and home care instructions. If the patient has improved, they can be placed back in the regular recall program with perio maintenance every 3 - 6 months. If the patient's condition has not improved, more advanced treatment or additional root planing may become necessary. Referral to a specialist should be considered and discussed if the patient is not responding to treatment.	• 40 - 60 minutes
Class IV & V- *Advanced Periodontitis* *and Refractory Periodontitis*	*Referral to a periodontist*

INTRODUCING YOUR PERIO PROGRAM TO PATIENTS

If you have never had a periodontal program in your practice, you may find that many of your patients will be surprised when informed they must go on a perio maintenance program. You may receive questions or comments like, *"Why didn't you do this before?"* or *"I've never heard anything about this. Why do I need this program when for years, I've only had to come in twice a year?"* Your patients need answers to these questions. Sample responses include:

- *"We've implemented this program so that we can detect and treat mild gum disease before any major problems occur and comprehensive treatment becomes required. Periodontal probing and charting is now a necessary part of every adult's regular hygiene appointment in our practice."*
- *"Dr. Michaels has always treated patients with gum disease when it appeared. However, with early detection for every adult patient, we hope to prevent and treat gum disease in its early stages before it becomes difficult to treat and more costly."*
- *"Dr. Smith has been watching your gum condition and has decided that the periodontal program would be the best course of action."*

Most patients will be receptive to your periodontal program if you take the time to communicate and offer explanations for your proposed treatment. Education is the key to acceptance. Visual tools are easier for patients to understand. For example: bleeding points with a toothpick or an intraoral camera to see calculus and red gums. Dental assistants and hygienists reinforce the dentist's treatment plan, but it is also important to train business assistants to answer the patient's questions positively and clearly when they are asked in the business area of the office.

TIPS FOR EDUCATING PATIENTS ABOUT PERIODONTAL DISEASE AND PROGRAMS

- Before the hygienist begins the probing and charting they should tell the patient exactly what they will be doing and why. The hygienist should inform the patient of the benefits of early detection and the new program offered in your practice.

- Always have patient education brochures about periodontal disease available in your greeting area. Although many patients are well informed, some have no knowledge of periodontal disease and subsequent tooth loss if left untreated.

- Patient education videos should be available to those with gingivitis or periodontal disease. If your patient is hesitant about the perio program, allow them to watch the video for detailed information. Visual tools are an important and powerful part of patient education.

- Computerized perio charting programs are excellent educational tools for patients. Computerized charting is also excellent for the dental practice. The chart should be taken before, during and after treatment so that the patient can see visible signs of improvement. Computer charting is faster and more efficient for the dental practice. An added benefit is that patients see computerization (namely chairside computerization) as a sign of an up-to-date, progressive practice.

- Give your patients a copy of the proposed treatment plan for them to keep. This can help them decide to proceed with treatment. The treatment plan also serves as a visual and educational tool along with a clear explanation of the fees.

- If your practice mails out a newsletter or if you have patient information brochures, you may wish to include an announcement of your new periodontal program. Explain the benefits and the procedures so that patients will have an understanding of it prior to their regular appointments.

- Hesitant or non-consenting patients should be sent a letter about the consequences of not completing necessary periodontal treatment. It is important that they know the consequences of ignoring periodontal disease. If your patient refuses necessary treatment, it is important that they sign the non-consent form to legally protect yourself (figure 6.2).
- Some patients will be uneasy about being treated for periodontal disease by a general practitioner. These patients should be referred to a periodontist for a second opinion. They can then be treated by the periodontist and return to your practice for regular preventive care appointments. It is the patient's choice.

The periodontal program should always be implemented for the patients' benefit. It should not be considered solely on the basis of increased production. Never push or force patients into your periodontal program if they do not want to accept. The only patients who should be in the periodontal program are the ones who require the treatment. To do otherwise would be unethical. I have heard of practices who implement this program and place many borderline patients in the program. The production increases and the practice sees great financial gain. But, eventually, the patients become discouraged about the fees and the treatment they feel they do not need. These patients leave the practice and seek another dentist. Your patient must need the treatment, be able to see improvement and an end to the treatment. If they don't improve, they must be referred to a specialist.

WORKING WITH YOUR PERIODONTIST

Sometimes a dentist is fearful of referring a patient to a specialist in case the patient does not return to the practice. In the majority of cases, this fear is unfounded. A good relationship with the specialist is necessary for the benefit of both practices and, most importantly, the patient.

If your patient does not respond to treatment or you are unsure about how to proceed, it is vital that you refer the patient to a periodontist immediately. This is where a good working relationship is necessary. The referred patient is still your patient even though you have sent them to the periodontist. Remember that the periodontist is there to treat a specific condition that the general practitioner cannot. Once the initial treatment has been completed, alternating maintenance perio appointments and G.P. appointments with communication between the doctors is in the patient's best interest. Discuss your periodontal program with your local periodontist.

WHERE TEAM MEMBERS FIT INTO THE PERIO PROGRAM

Each team member plays an important role in the success of the periodontal program. Although assistants or front desk staff may feel there is not really a place for them in the perio program, this is not correct. Each team member contributes to each and every aspect of the dental practice through communication and patient education.

THE HYGIENISTS' ROLE

In addition to treating periodontal patients, the hygienist has a role in the periodontal program.

1. **Patient Education**

   Patient education is one of the most important aspects of the periodontal program. Excellent instruction in home care is necessary for the prevention and treatment of gum disease. The whole idea of the perio program is to prevent, detect, treat and stop periodontal disease in our patients. Talking dentistry to patients is the best way to educate them. Never forget the visual tools. Give your perio patients the patient education brochures so that they can read up on their condition.

2. **Communication with the Dentist**

   The hygienist and the dentist are partners in the perio program. They must work together to treat each patient as an individual. No two patients will have exactly the same condition and so each must be treated accordingly. Communication about the patient's condition will result in the best possible treatment plan for that patient. The hygienist can document her visual findings for the dentist to confirm when he/she examines the patient.

3. **Talking Fees with Patients**

   There is no reason why a dental hygienist cannot discuss fees with the periodontal patients as long as they are comfortable doing so. They should not discuss financial arrangements, insurance, etc. The hygienist should have a list of the set fees chairside for each type of treatment and appointment. Once the patient has been diagnosed by the dentist, the hygienist can discuss the program treatment and number of appointments. The business team will discuss fees.

4. **Calling Periodontal Patients**

    Every hygienist should make an effort to call patients in the perio program to see how they are progressing – especially patients who have had a difficult perio procedure performed that day. Patients appreciate your concern and chances are, they will have additional questions which they forgot to ask about during treatment. Each call should take no more than 5 minutes and can be done before leaving for the day or during any down-time.

THE BUSINESS TEAM'S ROLE

1. **Patient Education**

    Every team member is responsible for the dental education of the practice's patients. When the patient comes to the business desk after an appointment, ask if they have further questions about the perio program or treatment. Usually, the dentist and hygienist have answered all questions but some patients will still have questions or they will want a confirmation of what was told to them in the treatment room. For this reason, each business person should have a solid understanding of dental treatments and the periodontal program. To help business staff with dental procedures, please refer to the Staff Treatment Cards in chapter 8.

2. **The Appointment Book**

    The business staff are in charge of the appointment book and are responsible for a smooth and productive schedule each day. The business staff help with the perio program by:

    *   Scheduling accurate time required for perio appointments
    *   Confirming perio patients
    *   Educating patients about the need to return for regular appointments (from the hygienist's note in the patient chart)
    *   Informing the hygienists of perio patients who cancel and do not re-book

3. **Meeting with the Perio Team on a Regular Basis**

    Staff meetings are essential to the smooth running of the practice. During your regular monthly staff meeting, comments and questions about the perio program should be discussed. If there are serious problems which show up in between monthly meetings, the concerned staff members should meet to resolve the problem(s).

THE ASSISTANTS' ROLE

1. **Patient Education**

   Once again, patient education cannot be stressed enough.

2. **Assisting the Dental Hygienist**

   There are many ways in which the assistant can be a part of the perio program. One of the best ways is to assist the hygienist during treatment. Duties which can be performed include:

   - Charting while the hygienist probes
   - Taking necessary x-rays
   - Taking and/or updating medical histories
   - Greeting, seating and dismissing patients
   - Cleaning and sterilizing rooms/instruments between patients
   - Assisting as needed

SUMMARY

- The hygiene department requires complete organization and an effectiveness rate of at least 75% for patient care.
- Ensure that you have considered all aspects of the periodontal program (costs, staff, chairs, training) before commencing.
- Ensure that you have organized your program (set fees, insurance, forms) prior to the commencement of the program.
- Make sure that your hygienists and other team members are thoroughly trained to perform the clinical procedures necessary for periodontal care.
- Don't be afraid to refer your patient to a periodontist if they do not respond to treatment or if you are unsure about how to proceed.
- Patient education is necessary to the success of any periodontal program.

AREAS OUR PRACTICE CAN IMPROVE UPON

NOTES

"Quality in a service or product is not what you put into it. It is what the client or customer gets out of it."

Peter Drucker

7.

MAINTAINING FINANCIAL CONTROL OF THE PRACTICE

"Great minds must be ready not only to take opportunities, but to make them."
Colton

Too many people tend to worry about finances rather than planning for financial success. Practice finances should always be monitored. This does not mean just regular bookkeeping and/or financial statements, but a true plan to monitor expenses and spending.

You must monitor finances in order to:
- maintain control of overhead expenses
- maintain control of spending
- maintain the organization of the practice
- chart your progress

AVERAGE PRODUCTION

On the whole, most dentists do very well with their monthly production and are able to generate a steady source of income. However, it is the expenses, overhead, extra spending and payables which decrease the profit margins in dentistry (or in any type of business).

Most dentists in a solo practice are able to produce approximately $20,000 to $50,000 per month. This figure rises or falls below average depending upon:
- The number of staff. A general rule of thumb is the more producers, the more revenue. Some solo practices with 2 or more hygienists and 3 assistants can produce up to $80,000 per month or more. Specialty practices may be higher.
- The number of dental chairs. Another rule of thumb: the more treatment rooms, the higher the production.

- The speed of the clinician(s) – both hygienist and dentist. Some dentists work very slowly, while others have greater clinical speeds.
- The rate of case acceptance. Far too many dentists are uncomfortable introducing comprehensive or elective dentistry for fear of rejection. Low case acceptance levels do not necessarily lower production, but they can stunt practice growth to a certain degree.
- The number of active patients. The more patients a practice has, the more patients they can treat and therefore the higher the production level.
- Scheduling procedures. In order to be productive, a practice must have a well-maintained, productive schedule with little down-time.
- The efficiency and effectiveness of the practice's business systems. A dentist can work at the speed of light but if the schedule is disorganized and there is no follow-up on missed appointments, pending treatment, insurance, predeterminations or collections, production is eventually affected.

MONITORING YOUR EXPENSES

To maintain a healthy financial position in dentistry, certain figures should be monitored on a monthly basis. In addition to monitoring monthly production and collection figures, practice expenses such as overhead, salaries, supplies, etc. should be maintained at reasonable levels.

Note: When I talk about percentages in this section, the percentage is of gross production, not gross collections. The majority of accountants and computer software programs calculate expenses through gross production. For the sake of simplicity, I have done the same (as long as your collections average 99%).

1. **OVERHEAD EXPENSES**

   The amount of your fixed overhead expenses should not exceed 55% of your gross production. If your practice is over by a few percentage points, this is fine as overhead can be lowered by increasing production or cutting back on some supplies. However, if your practice exceeds this level by 7% or more, you need to seriously look at where you are spending money needlessly. Or, you should be looking at scheduling and utilizing the clinical team more effectively. Overhead expenses (fixed) include everything that you must pay to maintain your practice:

- Rent/Lease
- Mortgage payments
- Staff salaries (incentive bonuses are not part of overhead expenses)
- Dental and office supplies
- Laboratory costs
- Telephone, fax, e-mail
- Bank charges
- Utilities
- Payroll and other taxes
- Legal and accounting fees
- Insurance
- Postage
- Equipment rental/lease

2. STAFF SALARIES

Staff salaries are a component of the overhead expenses but rate a category of their own. Staff salaries should not exceed 25% of your gross production. If your salaries fall higher than this percentage, either you are not producing enough for the number of staff you have or your staff are being paid higher-than-average salaries – more than your production figures can handle. Staff salaries include:

- Wages
- Income tax deductions and other payroll deductions paid to Revenue Canada (Canada) or the I.R.S. (United States). Staff salaries should not include occasional monetary bonuses or figures from a set incentive bonus plan.
- Spouses paid by income splitting should not be included. Only include spouses working in the practice.

3. OFFICE/DENTAL SUPPLIES AND LAB COSTS

I have included supplies and lab costs in one sub-section for ease in monitoring. Combined, this percentage should not exceed 25% of your gross production. Office/Dental supplies include:

- Printing costs for letterhead, business cards, envelopes, etc. This does not include promotional printing for newsletters, brochures and other marketing items. Any marketing items are not considered necessary to the maintenance of the practice.

- General office supplies such as pens, staples, clips, fax paper, etc.
- Paper supplies and patient charts.
- Dental supplies include instruments, accessories, gloves, burs, handpieces, pharmaceuticals, etc.

Your combined dental (7%) and office (3%) supplies should not exceed 10% of gross production. Laboratory costs are slightly different as they can reflect your case acceptance levels. Normally, the higher the lab costs, the higher the rate of case acceptance. Try to maintain your lab costs at 15% of gross production.

4. **OTHER EXPENSES – VARIABLE OVERHEAD**

This category of expense is entirely up to the dentist. However, the more money spent in this category, the less drawings for the principal(s). Be aware of expenses in this category.

- Dues and membership fees to associations
- Convention expenses
- Continuing education programs
- Incentive bonus plans
- Advertising
- Promotion and applicable production/printing costs for promotional materials
- Sales expenses
- Miscellaneous

For instance, if your practice had a gross income of $400,000, 5% would equal $20,000 – which is a fair amount to spend on extras. Supposing this dentist maintained his practice within the proposed guideline percentages, his profit/drawings would look like this:

$400,000	Gross production
less $220,000	Fixed overhead expenses at 55%
less $ 20,000	Variable other expenses at 5%
$160,000	The dentist can draw his/her salary from this amount.

Some dentists prefer to have a set salary (similar to other staff members) and this is fine. However, it should be based on actual practice figures provided in a yearly financial statement. (Your accountant should be able to give you assistance in planning a salary for yourself.) There is no point in taking home a $200,000 salary if your practice is going to have a net loss of $100,000.

See figure 7.1 for a sample Income Statement showing sample categories and expense ratios. Figure 7.2 provides a sample form you can use to monitor your practice's financial information.

MONITORING HYGIENE PRODUCTION

The hygiene production and other figures should also be monitored on a monthly basis. Hygienists are producers and as such, their production should be documented. Other figures to monitor include (see figure 7.3 for a sample form):

- The number of hygiene patients seen during the month. Monitoring the number of hygiene patients allows you to see how effective your recall program is and the average revenue generated from each patient.
- If you have an expanded-duties assistant who is trained to do prophies, their production level should be added into the hygiene production and monitored.
- The number of time units of down-time. It is vital that you monitor down-time to see exactly how many units are being lost due to cancellation, no-shows and improper scheduling. You can monitor the down-time for the entire practice on the Financial Progress Form (figure 7.2 – use column named "other").

CONTROLLING PRACTICE COSTS – NEED VS. WANT

Many dentists like "toys", objects or instruments which catch their fancy and once purchased are never used. Buying instruments and other toys which will seldom or never be used is a waste of valuable practice money which could be spent more constructively. If, however, the dentist finds something which the practice does not particularly need but would add another dimension to the practice (such as an intraoral camera), a "luxury sheet" should be used (see figure 7.4). This helps to plan for the costs involved and to set a target date for purchasing the "luxury" when the practice has budgeted for it.

FIGURE 7.1 SAMPLE: INCOME STATEMENT WITH EXPENSE BREAKDOWN

Gross Production		$545,000
Bank Loan	14,050	1. Overhead expenses
Legal/Accounting	7,390	$324,930 or 60% of
Health Tax	1,540	gross production.
Rent	35,500	
Telephone	4,230	
Utilities	7,850	2. Supplies/Lab Costs
Office Supplies	4,500	$93,635 or 17% of
Printing	4,540	gross production.
Interest - Bank	2,500	
Bank Charges	4,053	3. Staff Salaries
Insurance	5,872	$129,070 or 24% of
Postage	2,020	gross production.
Equipment Rental	8,880	
Dental Supplies	35,795	4. Other expenses
Lab Bills	57,840	$32,291 or 6% of
Staff Salaries	119,580	gross production.
Payroll Deductions	9,490	
Incentive Bonus Plan	6,375	
Dues/Memberships	2,400	
Conventions	5,780	
Continuing Education	4,530	
Advertising	3,703	
Promotion	3,483	
Miscellaneous	6,020	
Dentist Salary/Drawing	180,000	
	$537,221	
Net Income/(loss)	$7,779	

FIGURE 7.2 SAMPLE: DENTAL PRACTICE FINANCIAL PROGRESS FORM

NP - New Patients
NS - No Show Patients
Other - A Category of your choice to monitor

Month	Production	Collections	A/R Balance	Overhead		Staff Salary		Supply/Lab		Other Exp.		# NP	# NS	Other
				Total	%	Total	%	Total	%	Total	%			
January														
February														
March														
April														
May														
June														
July														
August														
September														
October														
November														
December														
Total														

FIGURE 7.3 SAMPLE: HYGIENE MONITORING FORM

Hygienist I Name:				Hygienist II Name:				Hygienist III Name:			
Month	Production	# Patients	T.U. D/T	Month	Production	# Patients	T.U. D/T	Month	Production	# Patients	T.U. D/T
JAN				JAN				JAN			
FEB				FEB				FEB			
MAR				MAR				MAR			
APR				APR				APR			
MAY				MAY				MAY			
JUN				JUN				JUN			
JUL				JUL				JUL			
AUG				AUG				AUG			
SEP				SEP				SEP			
OCT				OCT				OCT			
NOV				NOV				NOV			
DEC				DEC				DEC			
Total				Total				Total			

FIGURE 7.4 SAMPLE: LUXURY SHEET

Luxury	Total Cost	Monthly Cost	Goal Date	☑

INCREASING PRACTICE PRODUCTION

There are a number of ways to increase your production in dentistry, most of which have to do with organized and efficient business systems.

1. **EFFECTIVE AND PRODUCTIVE SCHEDULING**

   If your practice has the staff (two assistants) and the treatment rooms, double or multiple appointing can increase production, but only if handled properly. When double appointing, many business assistants make the mistake of scheduling two patients for the dentist at the same time. Unfortunately, the dentist can be in only one treatment room at a time. This is where the need for two dental assistants comes in. While the first dental assistant is seeing one patient, the dentist is in the other room treating a different patient with another assistant. A well-scheduled day utilizing the multiple-appointing method is shown in figure 7.5.

   Down-time results in lost revenue and therefore, it is in your best interest to eliminate as much down-time as possible.

   - When scheduling, never leave time units between patients, with the exception of clean-up time for the assistant and hygienist. If the hygienist is working with an assistant, the clean-up is allowed for in the time scheduled for patients (figure 7.5).
   - When a patient cancels, the appointment secretary must utilize a short call list to find someone who can come in on short notice.
   - Always confirm long appointments.
   - Follow up on all unscheduled treatment.

2. **YOUR RECALL PROGRAM**

   Effective recall programs are responsible for 30% to 40% or more of a practice's production. In addition, much of a dentist's comprehensive and elective dentistry comes from the regular recall patients. Therefore, an effective and organized recall program is a key factor to increased production.

   - A hygienist should see on an average day, approximately 10 patients. This can be accomplished only if you are scheduling the accurate time units required, not automatically 45 minutes or one hour. Some patients do not require scaling and may be treated within 30 minutes while others may require a more extensive treatment of 60 minutes. The hygienist must make a note on the patient's chart as to how much

FIGURE 7.5 SAMPLE: MULTIPLE-APPOINTING METHOD

Assistant I Time		
Assistant II Time		

	Dr. Room I	Dr. Room II	Hygiene Room
8:00			
8:10	Crown Prep	Emergency	Recall Appt.
8:20			
8:30		asst. clean up time	
8:40		New Patient Consult	
8:50			Recall Appt.
9:00		asst. clean up time	
9:10		asst. lab time	
9:20	asst. clean up time		
9:30	Extraction		Recall Appt.
9:40			
9:50			
10:00	asst. clean up time	Denture Adjustment	
10:10	Bridge -Prep/Imp		Recall Appt.
10:20		asst. clean up time	
10:30		Emergency	
10:40			Recall Appt.
10:50		asst. clean up time	
11:00		asst. lab time	
11:10			
11:20			
11:30	asst. clean up time	New Patient Exam	
11:40			
11:50			
12:00	LUNCH	asst. clean up time	LUNCH
12:10			
12:20		LUNCH	
12:30			
12:40	Amalgam		Recall Appt.
12:50			
1:00		Child Prophy	
1:10	asst. clean up time		Recall Appt.
1:20	Amalgam		
1:30		asst. clean up time	
1:40		New Patient Exam	
1:50	asst. clean up time		Recall Appt.
2:00	Denture - Imp		
2:10		asst. clean up time	
2:20		Child Prohpy	
2:30	asst. clean up time		
2:40	Amalgam		Recall Appt.
2:50		asst. clean up time	
3:00		asst. lab work	
3:10	asst. clean up time		
3:20	Bleaching		Recall Appt.
3:30			
3:40			
3:50	asst. clean up time		Recall Appt.
4:00		Emergency	
4:10			
4:20		asst. clean up time	
4:30	END		
4:40			
4:50		END	
5:00			END
5:10			
5:20			
5:30			
5:40			
5:50			
6:00			
6:10			
6:20			
6:30			
6:40			
6:50			

time is required so that the appointment secretary can schedule the correct number of time units.

- Preappointing is the best method for recall systems. Most patients will preappoint as long as they are guaranteed some type of reminder prior to their next appointment.
- The hygienist should make it a point to reinforce the dentist's treatment plan (if applicable) during the hygiene appointment. Educating your patient about treatment options and methods will lead to increased case acceptance levels.

3. **REACTIVATING PATIENT CHARTS**

Your patient charts should be reactivated on a regular basis to eliminate losing patients. Any patient who has not been in for one year or more should be called in order to get them back into the appointment book for a recall appointment or to complete necessary treatment. Reactivating charts should be an ongoing process throughout the year. The patients to call are:

- Patients who have not been in for one year or more.
- Patients who have not yet completed their treatment.
- Patients who have treatment pending.

4. **PATIENT NUMBERS**

Increasing your active patient base will increase your production. In the average solo practice with 4 to 5 team members, there are approximately 1,500 active patients. Each dentist should have at least 25 new patients per month. If your new patient numbers fall significantly below this figure, I would recommend that you implement some type of marketing plan to increase new patients levels in your practice. Please refer to Chapter 10 for more details.

5. **UNDERSTAFFING**

Being understaffed will stunt your practice growth. To be effective and productive, you must have the correct number of staff for the number of patients who are active in your practice. If your practice is producing $40,000 per month and you have only one business assistant, much of the follow-up administration work will not be completed in a timely manner. Your schedule will suffer and the stress level of the practice will be higher.

Some general rules for staffing include:
- One business assistant for each $35,000 per month in production
- One dental assistant for each scheduled dental chair
- One full-time dental hygienist for 1,000 active patients

An entire chapter has been devoted to increasing case acceptance. Please refer to Chapter 8 for more details.

SUMMARY

Financial success is definitely no accident, but neither is failure. We are responsible for whatever we accomplish or lose in life. We must plan for financial success instead of waiting for it to happen.
- You must have excellent, organized business systems for collections, payables and monitoring.
- You must have the right person at the front desk to discuss and collect fees.
- Your financial policies should be consistent and enforced.
- You need a competent and well trained bookkeeper or office administrator.
- You need an excellent accountant.
- You also need a bank manager with whom you can communicate.

AREAS OUR PRACTICE CAN IMPROVE UPON

NOTES

"Banks will only lend you money if you can prove you don't need it."
Mark Twain

8.

INCREASING CASE ACCEPTANCE OF ELECTIVE AND RESTORATIVE DENTISTRY

There is much more aesthetic awareness in the world today. Society's focus is on health with an emphasis on looking and feeling better. This is a "look good, feel good" generation. In dentistry, we must enhance our patients' understanding of their dental care. Educating our patients "dentally" is vital to heighten case acceptance of comprehensive or elective treatment.

Your dental team plays an important role in case acceptance as the attitude of your office and team will affect the potential of your production and case acceptance levels. Educating patients through skillful, knowledgeable communication will increase the acceptance of optimum care.

Even before beginning to think about increasing case acceptance, your dental practice must have the following set up and in place:

1. **An Excellent Dental Team**
   You must be properly staffed with team members who have a sound knowledge of dental procedures and techniques. This is true for the business team as well as the clinical team. Your team members must also be positive, professional and cheerful. Patients are more apt to accept comprehensive dentistry from a practice that promotes a high-trust, professional atmosphere.

2. **Organized Business Systems**
   Your administrative areas should be organized for ease in patient appointing, follow-up and quality care. All financial arrangement forms and policies should be in place and effective.

3. **Detailed Treatment Plans**

   Before making a case presentation, you must have a properly detailed treatment plan for educating the patient. Your plan should include options and alternatives as well as the necessary fees and number of appointments. If a patient is interested, they will ask all of these questions.

4. **Clinical Know-How for Difficult Procedures**

   Although most dentists are capable of performing quality cosmetic dentistry, there will be some procedures which require additional knowledge and hands-on experience, which can be gained at any one of a number of clinical seminars or through a dental school. The same is true of your dental team. They must be trained for new procedures and/or techniques.

5. **A Professional Atmosphere**

   Your entire office and team should promote the idea of success. People are visual and patients will judge a practice's dentistry by the look of the office, dentist and team. It is important that your office be professional-looking and spotlessly clean. You and your team must look tidy and professional. Dentistry is a health care profession and patients expect their dentist and his practice to look successful and professional.

6. **The Team's Dental Health**

   You cannot sell dentistry, especially cosmetic dentistry, if your own teeth are not in perfect shape. The same goes for your dental team. It will be more difficult to sell cosmetic dentistry if you do not have a great smile.

PATIENT EDUCATION

Patient education is probably the key factor to increasing case acceptance of optimum dental treatment. The higher your patients' dental IQ, the higher the acceptance of comprehensive treatment such as cosmetics and extensive restorative work. To focus on education, we must train our team to "talk dentistry." In many practices, most teams are friendly and caring, but 80% of the talking is social and only 20% is talking dentistry. Patients want us to be sociable and they want us to be friendly, but they also want to know about their dental care. They want to be educated about dental treatment and most important, they want us to listen to their dental needs and concerns.

Your entire team plays an important role in dental education.

BUSINESS ASSISTANTS

Every business assistant at the business desk fields clinical questions from patients. The patient may have just left the treatment room and will often turn to the receptionist for clarification on a procedure. Even though the dentist or assistant has just explained the procedure, the patient may need more information, so they ask your front desk team. This is why it is important that all team members be well versed in dental terminology, procedures and techniques.

- Allow your business desk team to observe procedures as part of their staff training. Observation will give them new insight into dental treatment which cannot be gained through a book.
- Spend extra time training your business staff in the many different clinical procedures available. Setting up a training schedule for a few weeks for observation will greatly increase your front desk team's knowledge. This information can then be passed onto the patient confidently by administrative staff.
- Use Staff Treatment Cards (figure 8.1) to help your business team gain new dental knowledge. Staff treatment cards detail, in layman's terms, different dental procedures, the number of appointments, how long the dentistry lasts, the advantages of the treatment and the general treatment cost. These cards make it easy for business staff to pass on dental knowledge to inquiring patients.

DENTAL ASSISTANTS

Dental Assistants have been clinically trained and should be well versed and knowledgeable about all types of dental procedures in a general practice. Assistants often find that patients ask them questions about procedures, new techniques, technology, dental fears, etc. Always ensure that your assistants are up to date on all current techniques in dentistry.

DENTAL HYGIENISTS

The hygienist plays an important role in patient education as they spend the most quality time with the patient outside of the dentist. A hygienist should educate their patients by:

FIGURE 8.1 SAMPLE: STAFF TREATMENT CARDS

PORCELAIN VENEERS

WHEN TO USE: For chipped, stained, damaged or malaligned teeth.

 # OF APPTS.: _____

PROCEDURE:
1. A small layer of tooth enamel is removed and an impression is taken of the teeth (the venners are made at the lab).
2. The teeth are acid etched and cement is applied to the surface. The veneers (tooth shell made of porcelain) are then attached and polished (Step 2 is at a second appointment).

DURABILITY: 4 - 10 years

COST: $_____

ADVANTAGES:
1. Looks very natural and camouflages stains, chips, etc.
2. Short procedure - usually two visits.
3. Quite durable and can be long lasting with proper care.
4. Improves the self-confidence of the patient.

- Instructing on home care. Even though this is a regular part of the recall appointment, the hygienist should expand on the dental talk for education purposes. They could discuss a new technique that the dentist has introduced, or new technology in the dental field: anything dental to raise your patient's awareness.
- Asking patients how they feel about their teeth and smile. Often a patient is more willing to discuss these things with the hygienist rather than with the dentist. Take time to communicate with your patients about their opinion of their own dental look. Ask probing questions and make a note of the patient's response for the dentist: *"Do you like the way your teeth look when you smile?"*

IN THE DENTAL PRACTICE

There are a number of ways to educate your patients in the dental office.

- Patient education brochures should be available in your reception area for patients to read. Nice displays for brochures should be used rather than having them lying haphazardly on a table.
- There are some excellent "Before-and-After" photo books available. These books should not only be in your greeting area, but also in your treatment rooms for patients to glance through. Visual tools are very important to selling dentistry.
- A tasteful bulletin board/wall for patient education is another excellent visual tool (not a cork board that has articles with pins stuck in them). I have been to offices that have a wall dedicated to patient education photos. The photos are usually framed before-and-after shots. At the top, you may wish to place a sign with wording similar to,

  "You don't have to be born with a beautiful smile to have one."
  "Ask our team how you, too, can have a beautiful smile."
  "Cosmetic dentistry is for everyone."

- Some patients may be hesitant about comprehensive or elective dentistry. If you have a video machine in the practice, there are some excellent tapes on cosmetic dentistry. The videos explain the procedures, showing before-and-after cases.
- The intraoral camera is an excellent visual tool for patient education and increasing case acceptance.

MARKETING YOUR COSMETIC/ELECTIVE SERVICES TO PATIENTS

Patient education is not the only way to increase case acceptance of elective and comprehensive dental treatment. You may also market your services to patients so that they are aware that this type of treatment is available.

- You can market your cosmetic services to patients in your dental newsletter. If you have an article about some cosmetic procedures (i.e., bleaching, bonding), you will generate interest among patients who do not like their smile.
- If you have recently taken a course on cosmetic dentistry, you should include a notice in your practice newsletter to create awareness.
- Your patient information brochure should have a listing of all the services that you perform in addition to general restorative and preventive dentistry. The more patients are aware of your services, the better the chance that they will ask about them.
- Your Yellow Pages advertisement can also be used to create an awareness of cosmetic procedures. This should be done tastefully. Please see the examples in chapter 10 on marketing.
- In some areas, it is permissible to market your practice through direct mailings. This usually takes the form of an envelope filled with local business offers. If your advertisement is tasteful and professional looking, then this type of marketing would be acceptable.

STEP-BY-STEP CASE ACCEPTANCE FOR NEW AND EXISTING PATIENTS

1. Enhancing case acceptance begins with the new patient examination or at the regular preventive care appointment. After reviewing the office policies and practice information with the business assistant (if a new patient), the patient is shown to a treatment room and the medical history should be taken chairside by a dental assistant. In addition to taking the medical history, the assistant can find out the patient's dental comfort level (on a scale of 1 - 10). The assistant may also ask questions such as:
   - *"How do you like your smile?"*
   - *"How do you like the colour/shape of your teeth?"*
   - *"Is there anything about your smile that you would like to change?"*
   - *"When was the last time you visited a dentist?"*

The assistant should document their conversation. At this point, the assistant can review the patient's dental history with the new patient (or the dentist, as some prefer). Basic questions of this type can be delegated by the dentist to the assistant. If the patient is in for a recall appointment, these questions can be asked by the dental hygienist.

2. The doctor will come in to do the examination and may (depending on the oral condition) diagnose their immediate concerns and/or basic restorative work and arrange an appointment to restore teeth. If the patient has expressed interest in cosmetic work to the assistant or hygienist, the dentist may take the time to explain procedures. Most new patients do not want to be confronted with a $4,000 case at their first appointment. If they mention it first, then by all means, go ahead. However, it is best to build a good relationship with the patient before introducing comprehensive dentistry. Fees should always be discussed before treatment.

3. If the patient requires treatment or has expressed interest in comprehensive care, a green, active tab should be placed on the patient chart. These tags are flags to the clinical team to promote the doctor's treatment plan next time the patient is in the office for a recall appointment. Some of your patients will choose to accept treatment immediately and others may wait. Patients accept treatment when they value and want it. It is a good idea to reassess patients every two years at a recall appointment. People's attitudes and priorities change over time and though they may not be ready for immediate treatment, they may want the treatment at a later date.

4. Selling and "unselling" dentistry is a problem in many practices. Some dentists are not comfortable with the word "selling". I am not uncomfortable with it because as a dentist you are not selling people something they do not need. Instead of "selling" you are actually:
    *   Educating patients
    *   Introducing treatment
    *   Listening to patient's needs
    *   Explaining and answering patient questions
    *   Informing patients of the consequences of not completing necessary treatment
    *   Being enthusiastic about dentistry
    *   Talking about the advantages of looking and feeling better

The way to introduce treatment is through education and listening to your patient's needs. If your patient needs comprehensive treatment or is not happy with their smile, there is no reason not to introduce treatment options. It is the patient's decision. However, patients must be informed of the consequences of not completing their treatment or refusing necessary dental work. Some dentists actually "unsell" dentistry. They put little "w's" over comprehensive treatment for "watch" or an "o" for "observe." What are you watching or observing? Does it need a crown or doesn't it? If you diagnose it, at least introduce it to the patient. Let the patient make the decision. If the timing is right, if they value it, if it's important to them at that time, then they will accept that treatment. *You cannot sell what you do not introduce.*

SUMMARY

- Listen to your patient's needs.
- Don't be overly conservative with treatment planning.
- Don't pre-judge a patient's ability to pay. Often the patients you least expect to accept dentistry do!
- It is quite difficult to introduce cosmetic dentistry if you and your staff do not have nice teeth.
- Don't exclude implants. Work with an oral surgeon and periodontist to introduce the option to your patients.
- Be proud of your dentistry.
- Keep your clinical skills up to date.
- Remember that a happy patient with a beautiful new smile will gladly refer to your practice.

AREAS OUR PRACTICE CAN IMPROVE UPON

NOTES

9.

SETTING GOALS AND PROMOTING TEAMWORK

Have you ever wondered why certain people and businesses reach their full potential? They are successful and seem to have accomplished so much. I don't believe it was by accident. I believe it was planned and the start of any plan begins by knowing what you want to accomplish and setting appropriate goals. We often have visions or ideas in our heads but it doesn't help if the ideas stay in our head. Goals need to be written down and a concrete plan must be implemented for success.

PRACTICE GOALS

For many dentists, practice goals are very important for planning. Practice goals can take many forms.

1. **PRODUCTION**
   For many, production goals are the most important area of the practice and to a certain degree, this is true. Without good production levels, there would be no practice.
   - When setting production goals, it is important to remember not to be unrealistic by setting unattainable goals. If your current production is $40,000 per month, it would be unrealistic to set a goal of $50,000 for the next month. Increase your production goal by $2,500 to $5,000 per month. If it is too high, you will demotivate yourself and your team by failing to reach your goal on a consistent basis. Set an attainable goal that is both realistic and motivating.
   - Set production goals on a monthly basis. You can also set yearly production goals but they are much harder to monitor.
   - Involve your entire team. They are the ones who will be helping you reach your production goals, so they should be aware of them.

- Write down your goals. This cannot be stressed enough. It is okay to have an idea floating around in your head, but if it is written down and shared, there will be more motivation to reach the goal.

2. COLLECTIONS

Collections cause problems for many practices. Unfortunately, there is no easy cure for collection frustrations.

- Set a goal to collect at *least* 95% of all production. There will, of course, be times when you have to write off an account but on average there is no reason why you should not be collecting 99% of accounts.
- Your team should be involved in collection goals as they are the ones that will be doing the collecting. At your regular staff meeting, make it a point to discuss overdue accounts and ways of collecting them. By keeping on top of your accounts receivable, you will decrease the need for constant collection calls to overdue accounts.
- Setting strong financial policies will figure prominently in your collection goal success. Remember that you are not a credit agency. Ask for deposits or for accounts to be paid in full at the time of service.
- Always document financial arrangements to decrease collection problems. If you have a commitment to pay in writing (with a signature), your chance of collecting the money increases significantly.

3. CONTINUING EDUCATION

Continuing education should be an important part of each dental practice. Once you stop learning, you stop growing.

- Look for courses which interest you professionally. Decide upon a course or courses for the year and budget accordingly.
- If you are taking a course as a team, decide together which one would best suit your practice. Upon deciding, you must set a budget and plan accordingly. An example would be to set aside $150/month for six months to pay for a team seminar in a different city or a national convention.

4. RETIREMENT

Everyone should plan for their retirement, dentist or not. You should not depend solely on a government pension when you are retired. There are plenty of options for pension funds.

- Set a year goal for when you want to retire.
- You must plan the sale of your practice in advance. If you have a partner or an associate, your decision may be easy. However, many dentists have solo practices and they should start to plan for the sale of their practice at least two to three years in advance of their retirement age. It is not easy to sell a dental practice in some areas. Therefore, much planning in advance of the sale is necessary so that you can retire on your target date.
- Keep in mind that the practices that sell fast are those that are productive, organized, well located and with a strong patient base. Your practice should be organized and financially secure anyway, but during selling time, a prospective buyer will be looking for these qualities.

5. **ASSOCIATES AND/OR PARTNERSHIPS**

If you are considering hiring an associate or taking on a partner, goals and plan setting will be important to your success. Document a date in the future when you you would like to have another dentist in the practice. Keep in mind that there is much research regarding contracts, commission, sales, buy-in amounts, etc. All of this should be well planned in advance.

6. **NEW PATIENT NUMBERS**

New patients are a vital part of the dental practice. The average dental practice should have at least 25 new patients each month for each dentist.

- Work as a team on a new patient marketing plan to increase your numbers. Plan which marketing techniques you will use and monitor your numbers accordingly.

7. **ORGANIZATION GOALS**

If your practice is unorganized, you must set time aside in order to sort out your systems.

- The most vital areas to organize include: financial systems, recall systems, accounts receivable and your appointment book. Set a target date for complete organization of your practice.
- Set aside one day per month (without patients) for cleaning up/ sorting out all files, paperwork, inventory, etc.

8. **LEISURE TIME**

Leisure time has become a luxury that many dentists cannot afford but really need. You must make the time for leisure activity and social time. You can set goals to:

- Cut back working hours on a weekly basis. For example, instead of working all day Friday, work until 1 or 2 pm instead.
- In the summer, shorten your hours for the week or take Fridays off.
- During slow seasons such as Christmas, take some time off. Often, people don't want to go to the dentist during the Christmas season as they are too busy doing other things.

You can produce the same amount of revenue in fewer hours by working more efficiently, not harder. You should have a well-balanced schedule utilizing the multiple booking method. See figure 7.5 for a sample.

This is by no means a comprehensive list. Our list is intended only to get you started on your goals. See figure 9.1 for a sample Goal Sheet to help you set clear goals and deadline dates.

MOTIVATING YOURSELF TO WORK TOWARDS YOUR GOALS

We need to understand that we have total control of our lives, and blaming people never gets us anywhere. If you get off track, give yourself a 24-hour mourning period; then get on with the business of reaching your goals. There is no real failure: the only failure comes from not bothering to try. Points to remember include:

- Dental teams are motivated by practice goals that are clear and realistic.
- Listen to those around you: are they positive? Surround yourself with positive people who encourage and motivate you.
- When work provides opportunities for growth, employees will be motivated.
- Making mistakes is part of change, growth and taking risks. However, make sure you do not make the same mistake twice.
- Do not procrastinate: "I'll work on my goals tomorrow". Do it now.
- Take the time to document your personal and business goals, have a positive attitude and remember that only a small percentage of the population reach their full potential in personal and business life. You are going to be part of that small percentile.

FIGURE 9.1 SAMPLE: GOAL SHEET

	JAN	FEB	MAR	APR	MAY	JUNE	JULY	AUG	SEPT	OCT	NOV	DEC
Production Goals												
Collection Goals												
New Patient Goals												

	DETAIL	DEADLINE	METHOD	BUDGET
Clinical Continuing Education				
Management Continuing Education				
Associate/Partner				
Retirement				
Leisure Time Goals				
New Office				
Office Deisgn				
Other				
Other				

- People often think about failure, but as my mother always said, *"There is no shame in trying and failing but if you don't try at all, then that is a shame".*

SUMMARY

- Set both personal goals and business goals.
- We should never settle for less than we can be.
- Fear is a limiting emotion.
- Never look back and say "I should have." All you have is now – take advantage of it.

AREAS OUR PRACTICE CAN IMPROVE UPON

NOTES

FIGURE 10.1 SAMPLE: CONSISTENCY IN MARKETING

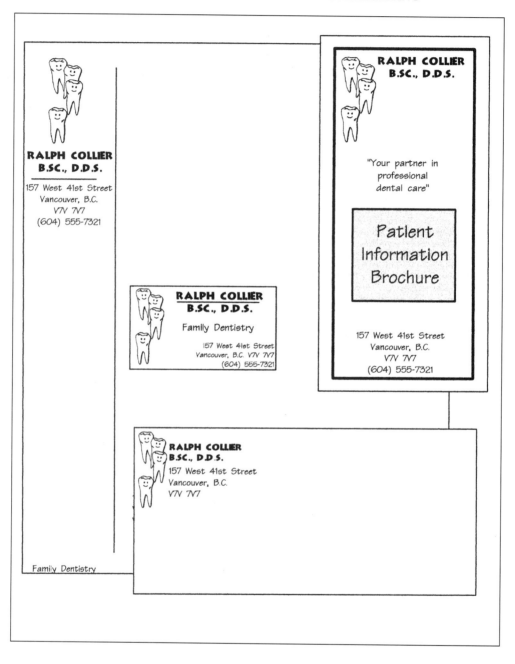

10.
MARKETING THE DENTAL PRACTICE

Consistency is the key to recognition in any business or industry, including the health care profession. Being consistent with your practice logo, letterhead, envelopes and business cards will give your practice the identity that it needs for patients (see figure 10.1). Our logo has changed 3 times over the years as our company developed in different areas. But on each occasion, my photo was used in each marketing item produced in order to maintain some form of consistency. Even with our new and final "world" logo, my photo remains as a source of recognition for clients and others in the dental community.

People identify symbols with things, people or places. For instance, the big yellow arches supported by a red sign is, for the majority of people, an instant recognition of McDonald's Restaurants. This is an excellent example of instant recognition for children who cannot read, but who read through the symbol of the arches. They know a McDonald's is nearby. Public awareness and identity is what you want to create for your own dental practice in a personal way.

Your logo or style should be printed on all outgoing items such as:

- Business cards
- Letterhead
- Appointment cards
- Confirmation postcards
- Patient education brochures
- Outside office signs
- Envelopes
- Newsletters
- Patient brochures

Designing a Logo for Your Practice

A logo is not an essential part of your marketing plan but it provides a source of identity to patients. Logo design can be done by anyone, you do not necessarily need a graphic designer to help you. The key is to keep it simple, easy to recognize and relevant to your practice or the title of your practice. Relevancy can also apply to your practice philosophy or to the character of the dentist. As you will see from some of the samples in this book, the logos match something about the practice.

There is no right or wrong with logo design. Your personal style and comfort level should be used. Of course, you must stay within the guidelines of your dental association or licensing body. For example, the R.C.D.S. in Ontario requires that you do not use certain words in marketing items.

Tips for Creating a Logo

- A modern practice should have a graphically modern business card.
- If you have an office motto, try to design a logo to fit your motto. One of my client's mottos is "Rising above the ordinary". All of his printed material has this saying, along with pictures of hot-air balloons. Hot-air ballooning is also his hobby (his practice is wonderful – far from ordinary).
- Make sure your logo is easy to read and understand. Far too many logos are filled with lines, pictures and words and no one is quite sure exactly what the picture is supposed to represent. "Busy" logos can also be difficult and expensive to reproduce.
- Remember that your logo has to be both increased and decreased in size depending upon how it is being used. Ensure that your logo can be enlarged and decreased without losing anything in the process.

If you are not comfortable with practice logos, you can still create an awareness through consistency in your outgoing material (letterhead, business cards, appointment cards, envelopes, newsletters, etc.). This means having the same type of print or the same colors. There are many attractive and professional fonts (type styles) on the market today. See below for samples:

Dr. Raymond Watkins   **Dr. Raymond Watkins**

Dr. Jennifer McDonald   𝔇𝔯 𝔍𝔢𝔯𝔫𝔦𝔣𝔢𝔯 𝔐𝔠𝔇𝔬𝔫𝔞𝔩𝔡

Dr. Saul Weinstein	**Dr. Saul Weinstein**
Dr. Marcia Barnes	**Dr. Marcia Barnes**
Cynthia Moore, R.D.H.	Cynthia Moore, R.D.H.

You can see the transformation from one type face to another. The names on the left look plain by comparison to the names on the right. Ask your printer for font samples and choose one that suits your personality and your practice.

PRINTING ON A BUDGET

Once you have designed your logo or chosen a font style, you are ready to go to the printers. Some tips for budget printing include:

- Choose one color of ink on colored or textured paper instead of having a multi-colored logo or print style. Printing in one color is the least expensive and you can achieve the color effect by choosing a quality paper stock. Also, the art and film work for multiple colors is much more expensive to produce than one-color art work.
- If you really want multi-color printing, try to stick with either match or process colors only. The more colors you include, the more expensive your printing and production costs will be.
- You can also choose a color and add "screened" colors of the same type. A screened color is just a toned-down version of the original color but gives the appearance of multiple shades. If using this method, you will incur additional charges in both film work and printing.
- Try to do any art work yourself. If your practice is computerized and you have an ink jet, laser jet or bubble jet printer, you can produce a good copy of your print style to the printer, thus reducing art work costs. Always take advantage of creative or artistic team members. This also adds an extra dimension to their job.
- Ordering in bulk is much less expensive than ordering for your immediate needs. If you don't plan on moving your practice or changing the name of your practice, your best bet is to order at least 1,000 business cards, envelopes and letterhead. A good print shop will counsel you on economies if you ask!

PROFESSIONALISM

Image is very important to a dental practice and in the health care community. Professionalism is necessary as your patients will see you as well educated, responsible and successful. Professionalism in marketing or design can take many forms. The cartoon caricature of a dentist on a business card is just as professional as a graphically designed logo on another. These are both professional because they give the patient something to identify the practice with – an aspect of the professional's character. By keeping your marketing professional, I am referring to keeping it consistent and tasteful – being yourself with style. Everyone is unique and what suits one practice may be offensive to another.

YELLOW PAGES ADVERTISEMENTS

A valuable marketing tool, Yellow Pages ads have become much more prominent in dentistry over the past few years. A good Yellow Pages ad can add to your new patient numbers – if presented professionally. In some areas, a dental practice cannot legally advertise in the Yellow Pages. Please check with your local dental association.

DESIGN

Ideally, a Yellow Pages ad should be designed by a professional (if in your budget) to make it eye-catching and creative. I recommend bold outlining for the ad so that it stands out from others and if your budget allows, color is an effective addition. You will find samples in figure 10.3 which can be used as a guideline to creating your own ad.

LOCATION AND SIZE OF THE ADVERTISEMENT

With the number of Yellow Pages advertisements now out for dentists, this is not critical. I recommend a medium-sized advertisement rather than one too small or one too large.

THE KEY TO SUCCEEDING WITH A YELLOW PAGES AD

The general idea of an ad is to create an awareness of your dental practice and to catch the attention of the type of clientele you cater to in your practice. Patients are looking for the following in a general practice advertisement (see figure 10.2 for a sample of an excellent G.P. ad):

FIGURE 10.2 SAMPLE: GENERAL PRACTICE YELLOW PAGES ADVERTISEMENT

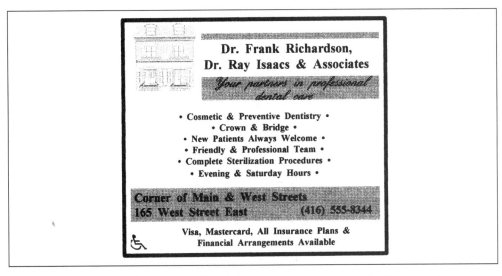

A. The type of dentistry offered (restorative, crown & bridge, etc.)
B. The location of the office
C. Infection control protocol
D. Financial information such as the acceptance of credit cards, financial policies, insurance information
E. If you accept new patients in the practice
F. If the ad looks "people-friendly"
G. If you offer emergency appointments

See figure 10.3 for additional samples of Yellow Pages advertisements.

BUSINESS CARDS

Today, business cards are necessary no matter what type of business you are in. Business cards serve the following purpose:
- They make people aware of the type of business you are in.
- They let people know where and how you can be reached.
- They create an awareness of you as a business person.
- They help to create an image of you.
- They can help to portray your image as successful depending upon the layout of the card.

FIGURE 10.3 SAMPLE: YELLOW PAGES ADVERTISEMENTS

Dr. Jane Jones

Dental Surgeon

555-1255
123 St. Michael Blvd.
Jonesville, Ontario P1P 1P1

General & Cosmetic Dentistry
We welcome new patients
into our practice

A general advertisement

JANE JONES, DDS

RESTORATIVE & COSMETIC DENTISTRY

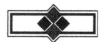

We welcome new patients
123 St. Michael Blvd.
Jonesville, Ontario P1P 1P1
555-1255

YOU DON'T HAVE TO BE BORN WITH
A BEAUTIFUL SMILE TO HAVE ONE

An advertisement to attract the type
of clientele you prefer

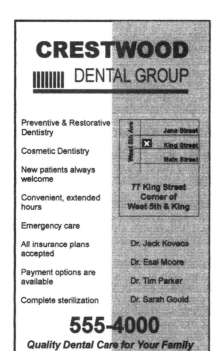

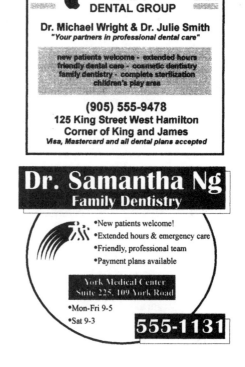

The idea of the business card is to create an image of yourself and your practice that you want to convey to your clients. You want to encourage the type of clientele which you cater to in your practice.

For example, if you want to promote your practice as restorative and cosmetic, the type of clientele you want to attract would be professional, middle-upper class, successful and the average age may be slightly older than in a general, family practice. These types of clients will be attracted to a professional, image-conscious dental practice. Therefore, your business cards (and other printed material) should be a reflection of the success of the practice and the dentist. A cartoon caricature of the dentist would not be appropriate for this type of practice. A professional, graphically pleasing, successful-looking card is what you require.

If you have a family practice, you want to appeal to the general public. These patients are from all age groups and from all social groups. They want a warm, friendly, professional atmosphere. They also want their dentist to be successful, but in a family-oriented, professional manner (see figure 10.4 for samples).

FIGURE 10.4 SAMPLE: BUSINESS CARDS

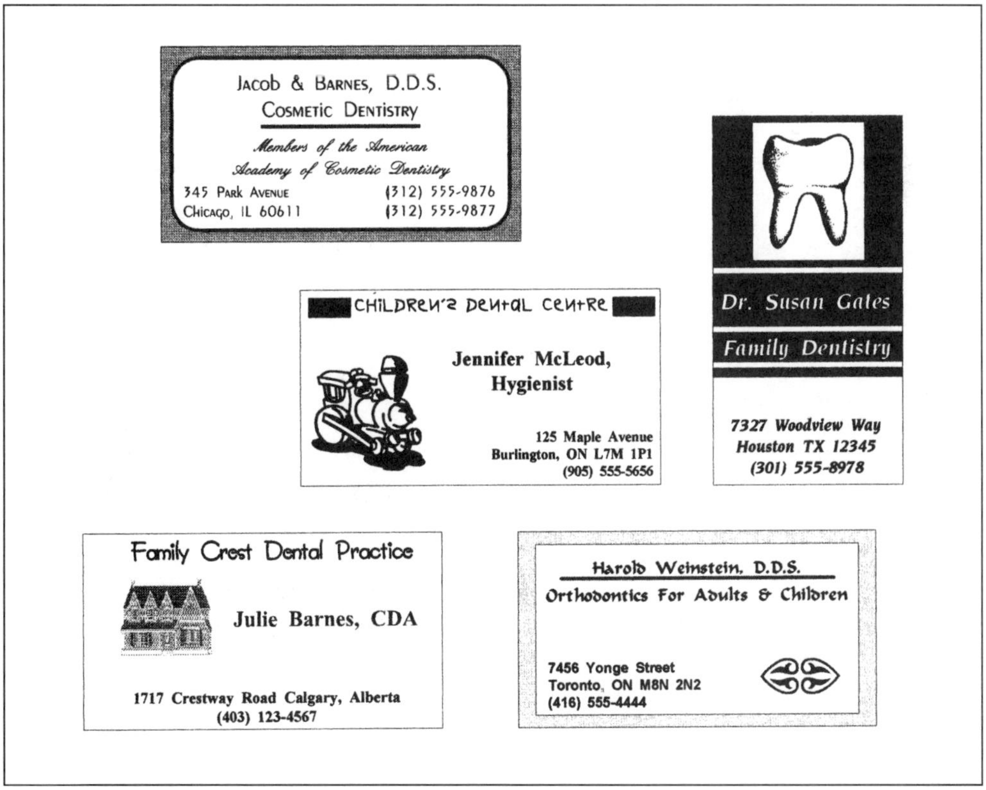

DESIGNING YOUR BUSINESS CARD

In Figure 10.5, the sample business card on the left is fine. However, it really doesn't say anything about the dental practice or the dentist. The key to marketing is to create an awareness for the public. To create an awareness, it is necessary to stand out from the crowd. The card on the left is similar to thousands of other

FIGURE 10.5

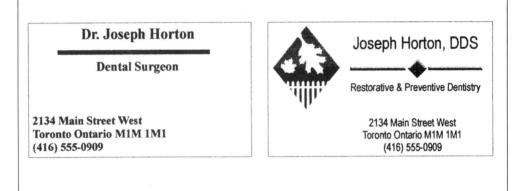

business cards – it does not stand out. The card on the right shows that the practice of Dr. Horton spends a little extra – he wants to portray a professional image. Therefore, by being slightly different, he has created an awareness of himself and his practice. If possible, you can use your name to identify with your logo. For example, a Dr. Hart could have a heart-shaped logo. See figure 10.6 as an example.

FIGURE 10.6

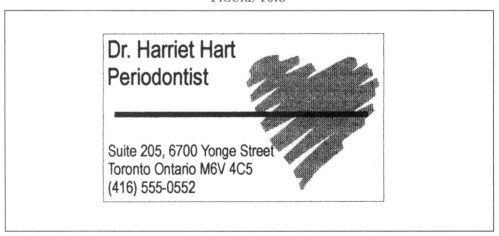

WHAT DO YOU DO WITH A BUSINESS CARD?

A business card is essential for everyone in your practice, but where do you place them and who do you give them to? Logically, business cards should be available at your business desk, in your greeting area and they are to be given to your patients. There are other places and other people to whom you can give a business card to generate interest in your practice.

LOCATIONS AND PEOPLE TO HAND OUT BUSINESS CARDS TO

- At local dental meetings – especially if you are practicing in a specialty office
- To tellers at your banking location
- To business associates
- To friends and acquaintances
- Socially, as you are asked what business you are in
- To stores near your practice
- Clinical team members should give their cards to patients; *"Mrs. Smith, if you have any questions about the treatment, please feel free to call me".*

STAFF BUSINESS CARDS

Staff business cards are great practice builders and make your team feel good about their positions in the practice. Staff can hand out their cards to existing patients and it lets the patient know who to speak with should they have a specific question for that staff member. For example, your hygienist can hand out his/her card to a patient while saying, *"Mrs. Smith, the periodontal program has been working very well for you. I can see that you've taken a great deal of care in your home perio care. If you have any questions at all, please give me a call and I'll be happy to answer them. Here's my card and the number you can reach me at."* This verbal exchange has let Mrs. Smith know that she is free to call at any time with questions and that she knows exactly who to speak with because she has the business card to keep as a permanent reference. Business cards are also great for a large front desk team who all handle different aspects of the business desk. The patient will receive a business card and know exactly who to speak with when they need any questions answered related to treatment, scheduling or finances.

Reasons for staff business cards
- An enthusiastic dental team are a great source for referrals.
- Cards make staff feel good about their positions and themselves.
- Your patients will know and remember staff members' names.
- Your patients will know who they need to speak with at your practice.

- They show staff that the dentist has confidence in them as an integral part of the dental team.

Staff business cards should always have the name of the dentist or the practice on the card.

THE OFFICE BROCHURE

An office brochure is an essential part of marketing, and adds a nice touch to your marketing plan. In addition to being a marketing tool, the office brochure is a valuable source of information for your patients. The brochure should be easily visible and available in your greeting area. The brochure should also be mailed to all new patients with a "Welcome to Our Practice" letter.

The brochure is divided into the following sections:

A. A welcoming paragraph to the patient. You may wish to discuss your practice and patient care philosophies in this area.
B. Office hours, address and telephone number(s).
C. Emergency treatment options and telephone numbers.
D. Practice policies, which include:
    1. Financial policies
    2. Insurance policies
E. Safety and infection control procedures.
F. Appointment protocol including late patients, cancellations, etc.
G. The services offered in your practice such as cosmetic dentistry, crown and bridge, nitrous oxide, etc.
H. Let patients know that you accept and welcome new patients and appreciate their referrals.
I. Your office logo and colors.

Optional sections (space providing):

A. History of the dentist(s) or the practice.
B. A photo of yourself and/or entire team.
C. A small map locating your practice.
D. Other available features for patients including play areas for children, headsets during treatment, movies for pediatric patients, etc.
E. An introduction of team members (I recommend this only for practices with little or no staff turnover). Or, a comment such as, "We have a highly trained, professional team," is nice.

Tips for Keeping Costs Down

A. Try to stick with a standard-size paper such as an 8¹/₂" x 11" folded twice. If a printer has to cut your brochure to a different size, it will cost more.

B. Try to keep colors to a minimum. Each color is an additional charge. A way to make your brochure look colorful is to use screened colors. Ask your printer about this.

C. Get at least 3 or 4 quotes on prices from different printers.

D. If you have an ink, bubble or laser jet printer with good software, you may be able to do the art work yourself and avoid charges from the printer for this service.

E. Keep the image area at least 1/4" away from all four edges of the paper. When printing all the way to the edge, this is referred to as "Bleed". To achieve this, a printer must use a larger sheet of paper and trim it to the actual size. This increases your costs.

See figure 10.7 for a sample office brochure. Feel free to copy our sample or use it as a guideline for creating your own brochure.

Promoting the Type of Dentistry You Perform and Generating the Right Patient Base

Dentistry, like all businesses, has many specializations; as a result, the need to market those specializations has become necessary. What you need to promote depends upon the type of treatment you wish to perform. As you can see below, there are a number of areas where you can promote your type of dentistry:

- In your office brochure
- On your business card
- In your Yellow Pages advertisement
- In out-going patient letters
- In an office newsletter
- In schools, daycares, senior homes, etc.
- To general practitioners if you are a specialist

The type of promotion for one general family practice may be different from another type of general practice, as one G.P. may specialize in cosmetic dentistry while the other specializes in preventive and restorative dentistry.

You must try to promote your dentistry to appeal to the type of patient you want to cater to. For instance, if you are a general practitioner who likes to perform some orthodontic treatment as well as general dentistry, your patient base

FIGURE 10.7A SAMPLE: OFFICE BROCHURE – SIDE ONE

Crinklewood Dental Centre

General & Cosmetic
Dentistry for all Ages

Caring Treatment
by Our Team of
Dental Professionals

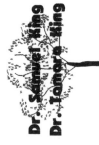

Dr. Samuel King
Dr. Tamara King

4545 Crinklewood Lane
Hamilton, Ontario L8P 18P
(905) 555-8777
(905) 555-8778
(905) 555-8779 Fax

Our Patient Hours:

Monday - Wednesday	8 am - 5 pm
Thursday - Friday	9 am - 9 pm
Saturday	9 am - 2 pm

Emergency Treatment

If you require emergency treatment during our regular patient hours, please call our office and we will see you the same day. If you have an emergency in the evening or during the weekend, please call our office answering service for the name and number of the dentist on call.

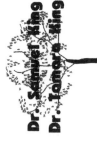

Crinklewood Dental Centre

We welcome and accept new patients into our dental practice. Please tell your friends and family about us. Your referrals are the nicest compliment we could receive.

Services Offered in our Dental Centre:

- General & Preventive Dentistry
- Cosmetic Bonding
- Porcelain & Laminate Veneers
- Crown & Bridge
- Full & Partial Dentures
- Teeth Bleaching

Other Services for Your Convenience:

- Play area for children
- Headphones for music during treatment
- Movies for children during treatment
- Nitrous Oxide is available

Infection Control & Sterilization Procedures

Infection control is an important part of any health care practice. For the safety of our patients and our staff, we observe the strictest guidelines available.

You will notice that all clinical team members wear face masks, eye protection and change their gloves between each and every patient. All instruments and handpieces are sterilized by our special equipment for every patient.

If you have any questions at all regarding our infection control policies, please ask any one of our team members who will be happy to answer your questions.

FIGURE 10.7B SAMPLE: OFFICE BROCHURE – SIDE TWO

Welcome to Our Dental Practice

Thank you for choosing us as your professional dental care team. You will find us dedicated to improving and maintaining your oral health. Our team members have all been specially trained to provide you with the best possible dental treatment and quality service. We look forward to working with you and your family.

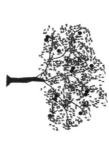

A Brief History of Drs. King

Both Dr. Samuel King and Dr. Tamara King graduated from the University of Toronto, Faculty of Dentistry in 1975. Together they opened their first practice in Stoney Creek, Ontario and in 1986, moved to this facility.

Dr. Samuel King enjoys cosmetic dentistry and has continued his dental education along this path. Dr. Tamara King enjoys family and preventive dentistry and attends many continuing education programs to continually update her dental skills.

Our Appointment Policies

Our appointments are scheduled exclusively for each patient. We try our best to run on schedule and ask that you do your best to be on time for scheduled appointments. If you are late, we may have to reschedule you for another appointment so that other patients are not kept waiting or we may perform part of the procedure originally scheduled.

All of our regular hygiene professional care appointments are pre-scheduled. This means that your next six month hygiene appointment will be scheduled while you are in the office for your current hygiene appointment. We will send you a confirmation card in the mail the month before your appointment and call to verify one or two days prior to your appointment.

We do not confirm any dental appointments (except pre-scheduled hygiene appointments). If you require a phone call to confirm your appointment, please ask one of our front desk team.

We ask that parents wait in our reception area while their child is having dental treatment.

If You Have any Questions...

Please feel free to ask any one of our dental team. You will find each team member knowledgeable about dental treatment, infection control and financial procedures.

Dental Insurance & Financial Policies

Please bring in your insurance booklet with you for your first dental appointment. If you have any insurance changes, please be sure to bring in the updated information for our front desk team.

We ask that all treatment be paid for at the time of service with cash, check, credit card or postdated check. Your insurance company will reimburse you directly. If a problem with your insurance arises, we ask that you call the insurance company directly, as dental insurance is a contract between your employer and the insurance company.

Financial arrangements are available upon request and our front desk team will be happy to discuss all options with you.

We will always discuss any fees with you before proceeding with any dental treatment. If you have any questions regarding dental insurance, financial arrangements, your account, etc. please do not hesitate to ask. We are here to help you.

Our Office Location

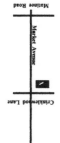

would be attracted to the following type of wording in a marketing presentation:
- Family and preventive dentistry
- Excellent infection control procedures
- New patients and emergency patients are always welcome
- Financial arrangements are available
- All dental plans accepted
- We accept Visa and MasterCard
- Play area for young children
- Crown & bridge and restorative dentistry
- Friendly, professional, knowledgeable dental team
- Sponsor of community sports teams
- Orthodontic treatment available by our specially trained general dentist
- Extended hours for our patients' convenience
- Multilingual dental team (this is best for large cities)

From this type of wording, your prospective patients will know:
- They are welcome in your practice.
- They can bring in their children without worrying.
- That you perform orthodontic, restorative and general dentistry.
- That your practice hours are convenient for working families.
- That you accept credit cards, insurance and payment plans.
- That you are interested in community events.
- That sterilization is very important in your practice.
- That they can count on you if they have an emergency.
- That your team is friendly and knowledgeable.

Some of the slogans for brochures, Yellow Pages ads (keep within your association guidelines), etc. that would appeal to this patient base would be:
- "Your partners in professional dental care"
- "Caring dental treatment in a professional environment"
- "A family practice for all ages"
- "Preventive dentistry with a difference"
- "Dentistry for the entire family"
- "_____ Dental Centre – Providing quality service and excellent dentistry"
- "General and preventive dentistry with a smile!"

The same rules apply to specialty practices – promote your services to the type of patient who requires your services.

INVOLVING THE DENTAL TEAM IN DESIGNING A MARKETING PLAN

To promote team spirit and enthusiasm for your dental practice, involve staff in your marketing plans. The more people involved, the more ideas will be generated. Below are some ways to involve your team.

1. **Ask for Team Ideas**
    Schedule a team meeting solely for discussing your new marketing plan. Each team member can think of ideas for marketing (either internal or external). At the time of your meeting, carefully weigh the advantages and disadvantages of each idea with the entire staff.

2. **Assign Tasks**
    Once you have made some decisions about your marketing plan and set an appropriate budget, you must decide who, what, when and how. I have included a chart in this chapter which shows how to record tasks. Tasks include getting different quotes from printers, buying new office decor, changing the wallpaper, designing a logo, writing the patient marketing letters, etc.

3. **Hold Regular Meetings**
    While designing and then implementing your marketing plan, it is a good idea to hold regular team meetings to check progress, prices, the meeting of deadlines dates, etc. Once your plan has gone into effect, you should also monitor your new patient numbers to see if they have increased and by how much.

4. **Take Advantage of Artistic Team Members**
    If you have a team member who is in any way artistic or creative, utilize their skills. This gives the team member a new and exciting challenge and your practice benefits from their skill, saving money by eliminating the need for a designer. Among the tasks an artistic team member can do are:
    *   Design practice logos
    *   Design an office brochure
    *   Design an office newsletter

- Design a Yellow Pages advertisement
- Give tips for office design

CREATING AN AWARENESS OF YOUR DENTAL PRACTICE – INTERNALLY

Marketing is not just external. You could spend thousands of dollars on an external marketing plan, but if you ignore internal marketing, you will have wasted your money.

THE OFFICE IMAGE AND ATMOSPHERE
1. Keep your office image professional and friendly.
2. Staff and doctors should always dress professionally.
3. Make sure that your office is spotless and uncluttered at all times – even during the day when you are working.
4. Make sure your magazines in the reception area are up to date and appropriate for the type of practice you have.
5. Ensure that the walls are always clean and the patient bathroom is spotless.
6. If you have a bulletin board, make sure it is not cluttered; keep it neat and up to date.
7. Always smile at patients when they walk through the door and greet them warmly – try to use the patient's name if possible.
8. Treat all patients with respect and kindness.
9. Promote a team spirited atmosphere so that patients feel comfortable when they are in your office.
10. Never speak negatively about your competition.

A KNOWLEDGEABLE DENTAL TEAM
1. All staff members should be well versed in clinical procedures.
2. All staff members should be able to describe each dental procedure should a patient inquire.
3. All staff members should be able to answer a patient's basic questions about dental treatment.
4. All staff members should know the advantages of different dental procedures.
5. The front desk team should be cross-trained for other reception duties in case one is absent for a day or two.

Team members should appear to be knowledgeable and intelligent at all times. Patients want to feel safe, secure and know that each team member is a dedicated dental professional who knows what they are talking about.

WORD-OF-MOUTH MARKETING AND REFERRALS

"There is only one boss, the customer. He can fire everyone in the company by spending his money somewhere else."

Sam Walton

We market ourselves each and every day whether we realize it or not. What we do (professionally), and how well we do it, generates talk about us. Word of mouth is an effective way to market a practice, complemented with a tasteful external marketing plan. Ask the following questions of yourself and your practice:
- What do we do better than our competition?
- What makes our practice unique?
- How can we improve our services?

In dentistry you must have excellent clinical skills combined with a knowledgeable, friendly team and above all, quality patient care. Remember that patients choose to come to your practice because of the entire team, not just the dentist.

THE 3 - 11 RULE

If you have quality service, excellent clinical skills and a friendly atmosphere, you can be sure that a patient will tell three other people about you and your practice. However, if a patient comes to your practice and is not please with the way you performed dentistry, a receptionist is rude to them or the office atmosphere is tense, then that patient will possibly tell eleven others of the negative experience in your dental office.
Make sure that patients leave your office:
A. Well informed.
B. Feeling special.
C. With all questions answered.

Cost-Effective Marketing

Many dental practices procrastinate over the development of a marketing plan due to cost factors. Surprisingly, you can market your practice on a limited budget – especially if you design your plan to take effect over a period of months. The key to controlling costs is to set a strict budget and remain within that budget. As you can see in figure 10.8, the budget for the sample marketing plan is both reasonable and cost-effective.

Cost-Effective Internal Marketing Ideas (From $0 - $100)

1. A smart, friendly dental team is a great asset. As you know, word-of-mouth referrals are a vital part of any marketing plan and a friendly, professional team will generate referrals.
2. A clean, spotless and uncluttered dental office shows patients you are organized and care about cleanliness.
3. A knowledgeable dental team who know the different procedures and treatments in dentistry shows patients your team is educated, trained and intelligent, creating a trusting environment.
4. Before-and-after photo books are great practice builders. They should be available in the reception area and in treatment rooms for patients to browse through. You can also create your own by photographing patients before and after treatment and using the photos in an album (with their permission, of course).
5. Holding elementary school tours of the dental practice. This is great education for the children and good for practice building. If this is not possible, you can volunteer to go to the schools and give a presentation.
6. Promoting your infection control procedures through a nicely framed notice in your greeting area.
7. Service, service, service cannot be stressed enough. Everyone on the team should be helpful and cheerful at all times to all patients.
8. Having those little extra patient services such as a separate play area for children (this only needs to be a small corner of your greeting area stocked with toys), headphones for patients to listen to music during long treatments, offering juice or coffee to waiting parents.
9. Holding patient contests generates interest in the practice. For example,

FIGURE 10.8 SAMPLE: MARKETING PLAN BUDGET SHEET

Marketing Idea	Month _Oct 96_	Month _Nov 96_	Month _Dec 96_	Total Cost
Internal Ideas				
Before & after books	35.00			35.00
Patient survey				
Name tags for the team				
Flowers for the office	20.00	20.00	20.00	60.00
Plants for greeting area		20.00		20.00
Framed pictures			50.00	50.00
Office paint			40.00	40.00
New wallpaper				
Office designer fee				
Team photograph				
Framed certificates				
Toys for play area		50.00		50.00
Headphones for music				
Cassette selection				
Juice/coffee station				
Magazine subscription	35.00			35.00
Coordinated uniforms				
External Ideas				
New business cards				
Staff business cards	100.00			100.00
Letterhead				
Envelopes				
Graphic designer fee				
Thank you cards	25.00			25.00
Birthday cards				
Yellow pages ad.				
Newsletter				
Office brochure		350.00		350.00
Sponsoring sports team				
New office sign			250.00	250.00
Patient letters				
TOTAL COSTS	$215.00	$440.00	$360.00	$1015.00

you could have a contest for children who have no cavities/fillings for the entire year. Their names are entered into a draw for a toy prize.

10. Play tapes or the radio in your greeting area and throughout the office. The music should be soft and relaxing. Hard rock is not acceptable for a dental practice. You want to put your patients at ease.

11. Make a child's first visit special. Take a polaroid photo of the child and dentist for the child's "growing up" photo album at home.

12. Special occasion marketing such as dressing up at Halloween. My former employer would dress up as the tooth fairy at Halloween. Some dentists wouldn't be comfortable with this, so keep it within your personal comfort level. (It was definitely fun!)

13. Patient surveys are an excellent way to receive feedback about your practice.

14. Make sure that your image and that of your staff is professional. Patients want a successful dentist and the way you dress and appear portrays your success. At all times, you and your staff members should appear clean, professional and happy.

15. Have lots of magazines and reading material for your patients. You should have a number of selections for most interest types: news magazines, children's books, women's magazines and general interest. Always make sure your magazines are up to date (within a couple of months). Buy magazine holders or always ensure that magazines are stacked neatly on a table or shelf.

16. Large picture books (animals, scenery, paintings) are nice for patients to leaf through. Not everyone likes to read, so an assortment of picture books is a great addition. *National Geographic* magazine is also excellent.

17. Have fresh flowers available in your office. Keep some in the greeting area and some at the front desk. Real flowers give an air of freshness to a dental practice. Never, under any circumstances, should you have plastic flowers in your practice. Nicely done silk flower arrangements are acceptable.

COST-EFFECTIVE EXTERNAL MARKETING IDEAS (FROM $0 - $100)

1. For computerized practices, use your computer to send out personalized patient letters such as:
   • Letter of appreciation to long-term patients.

- Letter to great patients (always on time, always cheerful, etc.).
- "Welcome to our practice" letters.
- "Thank you for your referral" letters.

2. Visit local daycares or kindergarten classes for a short presentation and hand out toothbrushes and stickers in a little bag. Don't forget to include your business card!

3. Hand out your business cards as discussed in the previous section.

4. Send out birthday cards to patients.

5. Send flowers to a new mom or to a patient who is getting married.

6. Keep the close parking spots outside for your patients and have staff members park at the back.

7. Make sure the outside of your building is clean, fresh and well maintained. This is sometimes hard if you are in a big office building. If you are in a small plaza or in a house, make sure the lawn is neatly manicured and the outside windows are always clean.

8. Offer to speak at a local high school's career day to discuss what it takes and what it is like to be a dentist, a hygienist, assistant or dental receptionist.

9. Plan an open house for your practice. You can offer juice, pop, and hors d'oeuvres. Mail invitations to patients and post a notice in your greeting area inviting your patients and their friends. A Christmas Open House and a Tooth Brush Exchange are great ideas.

10. On your business cards, confirmation cards, newsletters, brochures, etc. always have printed, "We welcome and accept new patients into our practice" and/or "We appreciate your referrals."

11. At Christmas, call a patient who is struggling financially and has tried to pay off their account. Write off their debt: "Our gift to you."

THE INTERNET: ADVERTISING FOR THE FUTURE

The internet offers an excellent way to market your practice as evidenced by the increasing number of dentists who advertise their practice and services on the World Wide Web (WWW). To accomplish this, you will need a computer, a modem, HTML (hyper text mark-up language) software and an internet access provider. The WWW comprises thousands of business and personal home pages, also called web sites. These home pages can be for personal, fun or business use.

A server (internet service provider, ISP) may provide free or minimal-cost home pages for their clients.

The costs for advertising on the internet vary.

1. You will need a telephone line to access the internet. You could use one of your business lines or a private line but keep in mind that every time you are on the internet, your telephone line is busy. If you have a computer in your home, you may prefer to access the internet from there.

2. You will need an account with an ISP (internet service provider). Costs for these accounts range between $10 and $50 or more per month depending on the number of hours spent on the internet. E-mail access is generally provided with the accounts, as is the software necessary for moving around on the internet (browsers).

3. HTML software will be necessary if you are going to write your own business advertisement. This software is available at computer stores everywhere. It is also available as freeware or shareware for downloading over the internet. If you do not wish to write your own advertisement or have no idea how to do it, there are many companies now available who specialize in creating HTML documents (also called Web Page Designers) for clients. Check with your ISP for referrals. Many of these companies also advertise on the internet. There will be a fee for this service.

4. You may have to pay your ISP for your web site. Currently, some of the smaller, local ISP offer free web sites to clients.

5. If you have an e-mail address but do not wish to have a web site, there are dental services on the internet which provide listings and descriptions of dentists and dental practices worldwide. Some services provide the listing free of charge.

For those dentists or dental staff members who already have access to the internet, I recommend that you use one of the search engines (search "dentists" or "dental") to see sample pages of dentists who advertise their practice on the WWW. Keep in mind that you must contact your state/provincial association to ensure that internet advertising is legal for dentists in your area.

The benefits of access to the internet are almost limitless. Already there are many worldwide, national and local dental associations, dental schools, dental magazines, dentists, continuing education seminars and reference areas on the internet. There are newsgroups and mailing lists dealing strictly with dental issues, techniques and practice concerns. All of this information is at your fingertips.

With the millions of people who surf the internet, this is an advertising chance you shouldn't pass up. Please e-mail our company at **ajupp@netaccess.on.ca** to view our web site on the internet. We will send you a reply with our current URL (location of our web site).

NEWSLETTERS IN DENTISTRY

A patient newsletter is designed specifically for your patients. The objectives of a patient newsletter are:
- To generate more business and referrals from existing patients.
- To give your patients access to information about dentistry, choices in treatment and about your dental practice.
- To reinforce the importance of regular, continuing, professional care.
- To increase the trust and loyalty of existing patients (*"Our dentist keeps us informed..."*).
- To enhance your community image.

Dentistry is filled with more media coverage than ever before. For this reason, the patient newsletter is an excellent way to allay patient fears about some of the following issues:
- Radiographs
- Infection Control
- Mercury
- Fluoride

In addition, your newsletter can be filled with any of the following types of articles:
- The services offered in your practice.
- Your office hours – especially if they change from winter to summer hours.
- A biography on the dentist.
- Staff happenings and patient happenings.
- Promote patient contests within your dental practice.
- Discussing new treatment available.
- Discussing new dental technology available.
- Photographs of your staff and practice.
- New continuing education programs you have recently attended.
- Different types of restorations (e.g., bonded amalgam or composite).

- Orthodontics for adults as well as for children.
- Caring for baby's teeth (baby bottle syndrome).

The list is practically endless. There are so many ways to fill a newsletter in dentistry. The only thing you have to watch for – when writing a clinical article – is not to become too technical. Keep it in easy-to-read layman's terms.

NEWSLETTER SETUP AND DESIGN

You must decide whether your newsletter will be issued monthly or quarterly. A quarterly frequency is more cost-effective as it will be issued four times per year as opposed to twelve. Twice yearly is also effective.

A newsletter must have the following qualities and characteristics:
- Your office logo and motto (if you have one).
- A heading or masthead unique to your practice.
- A newspaper-like design – either two or three columns.
- Some pictures are always pleasing. Use either clip art or photos of your practice, you or your team.
- Interesting articles written in layman's terms for your patients.

Please see figure 10.9 for a sample Newsletter Setup.

It is not necessary to produce a four-page newsletter. A two-page newsletter works very well for most practices and is much more cost-effective. If your practice is computerized with a bubble, ink or laser jet printer, you can produce your own two-page newsletter in your practice. You can print it directly from your printer in black ink and photocopy onto a colored paper.

Many companies provide newsletter services. They can incorporate your logo and articles into their own setup or you can choose articles from their abundant listings. The cost for newsletter services can be quite reasonable and most companies do a professional-looking job.

There are constantly changing rules and regulations with all dental societies worldwide related to marketing and restrictions. Always check with your association to keep within guidelines.

FIGURE 10.9 SAMPLE: NEWSLETTER SETUP

The Dental Gazette

115 Vantage Avenue
Halifax, NS B6F 6B6
(902) 555-8878 Telephone
(902) 555-8887 Fax

Taking Care of Baby's Teeth

Taking extra care with your baby's new teeth will help your baby to keep his teeth for a lifetime. New mothers should be aware of a dental problem called, "Baby Bottle Syndrome." When you give your baby a bottle of juice during nap times or during the night, the acid from the juice is left on the baby's new teeth. This acid, if left on the teeth, will eventually cause damage to the baby's primary teeth. It is very important that you brush your baby's teeth on a regular basis and avoid giving him/her juice when it is time to nap.

Once your baby's teeth have erupted, they can be brushed with a very soft and small toothbrush. We have some available in our practice for you to keep. There is no need to use toothpaste as the baby cannot spit it back out. Brushing with water will help to remove any soft deposits (plaque) on the teeth and thus avoid a build up of tartar and eventual tooth decay.

When your child is one or two, he will probably want to brush his teeth himself. This is fine as long as you have brushed his teeth for him first.

Proper dental care, from the first eruption of baby teeth, will ensure that your child will keep his teeth healthy and clean for a lifetime.

Our New Office Hours

Summer:
June 1 until Aug. 31

Monday	9:00 - 5:00
Tuesday	9:00 - 7:30
Wednesday	9:00 - 5:00
Thursday	9:00 - 5:00
Friday	9:00 - 1:00

Winter

Monday	8:30 - 7:30
Tuesday	9:00 - 3:00
Wednesday	9:00 - 5:00
Thursday	8:30 - 7:30
Friday	9:00 - 5:00
Saturday	9:00 - 1:00
	Alternate Saturdays

Dear Patients,

Welcome to the 5th installment of our bi-annual newsletter. We hope that the information provided has been educational and interesting for you.

Please make note of our new office hours for the summer. We are remaining open one evening per week for your convenience. Have a wonderful summer with family and friends.

Questions?

We are available to answer any and all of our patients' questions regarding treatment, insurance and fees.

Meet Our Team Members

Dr. Emmanuel Plania received his degree in dentistry in 1982 from Dalhousie University here in Halifax. He has been practicing family dentistry on Vantage Avenue since 1984.

Gloria Jacobs is our Office Coordinator who has 23 years of experience in the dental field. She has been with our practice since 1985.

Michelle Ledoux, our Business Assistant graduated from Dalhousie University and has been a valued team member since 1992.

Leslie Glodden, our dental hygienist comes to us from George Brown College in Toronto. She has been on our team since 1989.

Our newest team member, Daliah Ing is a certified Dental Assistant. Daliah has been a team member since 1995.

Jennifer Seddes, a certified Dental Assistant, on our team since 1991, brings to us 17 years experience in dentistry.

I would like to thank all of my staff for doing such a great job every day of the year. You are all valued team members. Look for a new addition to our team in the Fall of 1996.

AREAS OUR PRACTICE CAN IMPROVE UPON

NOTES

SUMMARY

After reading this book, I would encourage all dentists to plan a team meeting to share any new ideas and to generate enthusiasm for positive change.

In 1985, when I started my business, many people said things to me such as, "It won't work" or "Who will pay to go to your seminars?". Obviously, I didn't listen to those people; I listened instead to those who encouraged me, believed in me and could foresee the results.

As my company grew, we changed directions many times with new plans and new ideas. Many of our ideas were successful; some were not. Was it easy? Absolutely not! But it was worth all that I have experienced – stress, frustration, disappointments, results, profit and personal reward. Often, we felt as if we were on a roller-coaster ride. Eventually, with careful planning and motivation and a few wrong turns along the way, I am proud to have had the opportunity to lecture internationally and to have met so many wonderful people. It was well worth the effort from myself, my team and my family.

Many of you who have attended my lectures will notice that there is not too much humor in the book (I love to inject funny stories in seminars). Because I focused so much on facts, systems and communication, I never found the time to add in the fun stories. I have, however, already decided to write a third book, full of humor and the funny things that happen in dentistry. Nevertheless, dentistry is a serious business. Hopefully, with a new, strong business plan, you will begin to see the rewards from all of your hard work and together, reach your new goals and continue to find increased personal success and happiness.

I had asked some of my clients to send me a nice, inspiring quote for one of my books. The following quote was sent to me by one of my favorite clients, Dr. Ronald Ramsay. He is one of the most wonderful people I have ever met – a truly excellent dentist, kind, generous, caring and most importantly has a great sense of humor. When he first sent his quote, I thought it was negative and he had sent it as a joke. After reading it over a few times, I realized there was much truth to it. (Ronnie, thank you for taking the time to send me a quote)

Some people are unreasonable, illogical and self-centered – love them anyway.
The good you do today will be forgotten tomorrow – do good anyway.
Honesty and frankness make you vulnerable – be honest and frank anyway.

People favor underdogs but follow only top dogs – fight for some underdogs anyway.
Give the world the best you've got – anyway.

(author unknown)

If we all continue to do the best we can do, in all circumstances – even when we feel unappreciated – the world will be a better place.

I hope you will find my books helpful. I believe I have given you "the best I have to give!"

Anita Jupp
March, 1996

INDEX